Maximized
Metabolix™

A diet based on hormones and desserts

The Evidence is in:
Lose weight
Get healthy
Defy aging

Dr. Ben Lerner

NY Times, USA Today and Wall Street Journal
Best-Selling Author

With contributions from experts in the field of nutrition

EXPERT CONTRIBUTORS AND SCIENTIFIC EDITORS

Karen Vieira, PhD - Research, editing, and scientific review of all materials.

Peter Huth, PhD - Expert contributions on dairy.

The Med Writers - PhD-level scientific review of all materials.

William E. M. Lands, PhD - Author of Fish, Omega-3 and Human Health, Second Edition and the www.fastlearner.org/omega3-6balance.htm. Provided scientific review of fatty acids.

Judith Brown, PhD - Provided consulting on the curriculum outline.

Dr. Joel Villeneuve - Scientific review of all materials and contribution in the area of supplementation and metabolic testing.

Donna Marlor, BSN, MA, RD, CCSD - A sports nutrition expert working with the US Olympic Education Center. Provided carbohydrate metabolism and fitness content. donnamarlor. com.

Franziska Spritzler, RD, CDE - Nutritionist for the VA and writer for the American Diabetes Association. Provided carb conscious meal plans and recipes. lowcarbdietitian.com.

ACKNOWLEDGEMENTS

This book is written with and for the Maximized Living doctors and health care providers all over the world. They help to create, as well as study and master, these materials for the purpose of transforming and saving of thousands, and, ultimately, thirty-four million lives.

Special thanks to my wife, Dr. Sheri Lerner, who puts up with me and supports me during the research, writing, rewriting, and sweat that goes into these books. She, along with my children, Skylar, Nicole, and Cael, inspire me to eat and live this way so I can be here for them and spread this important information to other families.

CONTENTS

Critical Concepts of Maximized Metabolix
The Results Will Sound Almost Unbelievable

I was named after my grandfather that I never met. By the time I was eleven years old, all of my grandparents had died. My kids never met my dad. Sadly, he too had died before they were born.

Before I was thirty, I was having serious back and knee pain that I blamed on fifteen years of football, heavy weights, and wrestling. I was also having severe stomach and digestive issues since the age of eighteen from an anti-inflammatory drug. By all measures, I seemed headed down the same road as my forefathers.

I achieved my nutrition degree with hopes of finding a solution. But the low-fat, high carb guidelines we were following weren't doing me a gram of good. Then I made the switch. I changed to the type of eating and supplementation plan I will share with you in this book.

Now, at forty-seven, I am stronger, without pain, and in far better shape than when I was competing as an Academic All-American Wrestler in college. While I couldn't run by the time I was in my late twenties, I now do marathons and Ironmans. I am five pounds lighter than I was as a teenager.

The concepts presented here are far from an experiment of one, however. I can only write this book because I work with hundreds of doctors from around the world that provide the living laboratory for this work. Due to eating this way, the majority of them and their patients are seeing what almost seems like a miracle. But it's not a miracle—it's simply the way to eat to work with and not against your body's metabolism.

The average doctor's clinic implementing these solutions has photos of patients who take those standing next to their old "big pants" that they wore a half dozen or more sizes ago photo. It's so common for patients to lose twenty–thirty pounds or more in our offices, that it's almost mundane for us now. We expect it.

We also expect something even more exciting than the dropped pounds. There are seemingly endless numbers of people who fill up our throw-away drug bins as their symptoms and diagnosed illnesses disappear along with the weight.

I know it can seem like hype or hyperbole to say you can "defy aging." But it may honestly be the best way to describe how so many people I know and work with are living today. You've heard of forty being the new thirty, but we're seeing that fifty is the new thirty. Maybe even the new twenty.

It's simple and it works. If you don't believe me, just try it. Thousands of others have, and if they can do it—you can do it!

The Easiest Non-Fad Diet and Nutrition Book You'll Ever Digest!

This is decidedly a fat-focused, low-carb, evidence-based book. After many early years of teaching—and living—low-fat eating, the results weren't there. Now, with the strategies we'll show you here, my patients, family, and I, personally, have seen great benefits both clinically and physically—and the science is here to support it.

 I'm not opposed to other plans necessarily. Anything that moves you away from processed foods and junk and towards whole, natural foods is a step in a very positive direction. I was actually a vegetarian for several years after one of my nutrition teachers made me afraid of meat. I know firsthand how easy it is to upset vegetarians with a non-carb-based plan, but the good news is that they can't punch very hard, so I'm safe.

Where Does Good Health and Nutrition Information Come From?

I received my degree in nutrition in 1991. Not wanting to fall behind or be a nutritional has-been, I've read thousands of books, journals, articles, gone to seminars—you name it. With nutrition still something of a new field, it's been fascinating to watch the science of nutrition mature to where it is today.

Because nutritional science is still relatively young, many, many, many outdated theories still exist and get written up in the latest books. What's most important to you is that you get the most current, correct information. Which is why I'll share nothing here that's not only evidence based, but has worked on thousands and thousands of our patients around the world.

Together with our Maximized Living doctors, we work with Olympic, National Football League, Major League Baseball, Major League Soccer, and professional fighting athletes and take care of many famous people. As importantly, we take care of individuals just like you and me, from babies to centenarians. In other words, if you read it here, it's been cited in the world's leading scientific journals and it's worked on real people.

Life isn't lived in a vacuum. While nutrition is an incredibly important factor in health, I'm not going to say it's everything. While this book focuses almost solely on nutrition, Maximized Living has 5 Essentials:

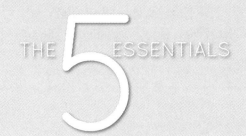

THE 5 ESSENTIALS

 Essential #1 – Maximized Mind *(knowing what it takes to experience real health and the mental skills to carry it out)*

 Essential #2 – Maximized Nerve Supply *(a healthy spine and nervous system)*

 Essential #3 – Maximized Quality Nutrients *(the Nutrition Essential)*

 Essential #4 – Maximized Oxygen and Lean Muscle *(the Exercise Essential)*

 Essential #5 – Minimized Toxins
Each of these Essentials work together to keep your cells in optimal shape and your body functioning at its highest levels. If you only focus on one of these Essentials, such as exercise, you are leaving out other core elements that keep your body healthy.

 This book is primarily about **Essential #3: Maximized Quality Nutrients**. Only read this book if you're trying to become the healthiest you've ever been, stay that way, lose weight, reboot your hormones, reverse inflammation, maximize performance, and/or defy aging. Because that's what it's done in my life and the lives of countless others.

You'll be happy to know that there's no deprivation to this way of eating. At least, not really. Any way you slice it, a slice of real New York-style pizza, New York-style cheesecake, and all of the other foods they make in New York that can kill you, those are the ones that taste best. On the other hand, we've got pizza, we've got cheesecake, and we've got nearly every other kind of junk food you can imagine.

We just do it Maximized Metabolix style. You'll find recipes here that give you a solid eighty-five–ninety percent of the pleasure with none of the guilt, cardiovascular disease, or weight in your buns and thighs.

We call it a "Diet based on desserts" because you can eat our desserts all of the time since they're actually made of ingredients that help and don't hurt your chances of reaching your health, fitness, and longevity goals. These foods taste great and make your gut and your butt smaller—and can help keep them that way.

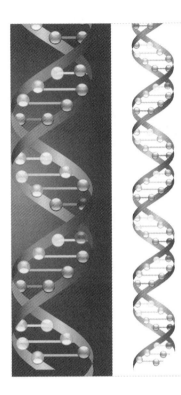

What is Metabolix?

In a nutshell, Metabolix is maxing out your metabolism. Your metabolism isn't simply how many calories you burn per hour. Your metabolism is your system of metabolics or physiology. It's your brain, nervous system, glands, and the chemicals and hormones they create. If this system is functioning at its max, you experience wellness and the kind of fat-burning, muscle-building metabolism you're looking for—without creating nasty by-products like insulin resistance, inflammation, triglycerides, and atherosclerosis, early aging, and disease.

The vast preponderance of real nutritional results is not based on calories, amounts of food you're eating, or going low fat. Weight loss, health, and anti-aging eating have more to do with hormones than with calorie-counting. That concept will make more sense to you once we're finished—and it will easily translate into a diet you tailor-make to suit your needs.

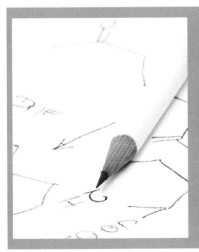

THE MAXIMIZED METABOLIX FORMULA
$$= H_2A_2$$

My college Chemistry 101 teacher used to call me a "one-armed bandit." In other words, I always simply wanted to know the formula. As complex as your physiology is, to achieve Maximized Metabolix, there are a few simple steps you can take to reboot your hormones, lose the weight, and slow down an aging process that may be galloping, rather than walking, you through the Valley of the Shadow of Death.

THE MEANING OF THE FORMULA

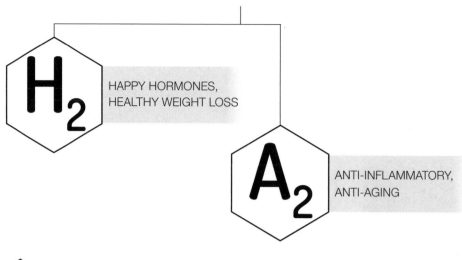

H₂ HAPPY HORMONES, HEALTHY WEIGHT LOSS

A₂ ANTI-INFLAMMATORY, ANTI-AGING

The Path to Happy Hormones
When you have Maximized your Metabolics, your hormones are working for you, not against you.

Healthy Weight Loss
To lose weight in a healthy way and without suffering and deprivation, you need, in addition to rebooted hormones, to become a fat burner and not just a sugar burner.

It's Better not to Burn out or Fade Away
Inflammation and oxidation—these are the metabolic terms of old age. They make cholesterol harmful, damage joints and arteries, and cause cellular stress that leads to chronic disease. And that's just for starters. When you're eating the right way, burning more fat than sugar, and balancing your hormones, you can slow or even reverse these problems. While being alive and living on earth will mean you have to endure some inflammation and oxidation, we'll help you minimize their effects as much as possible.

The Three Easy Steps to H₂A₂

The Western diet and many of the medical and governmental dietary protocols out there will make you age quickly and die fast. I don't have to tell you this: everyone knows that the nutritional impact on disease, aging, and early death is epidemic.[1]

The Maximized Metabolix Formula has three simple steps to take and a choice of two plans you can follow to suit your needs, desires, wants, and conditions:

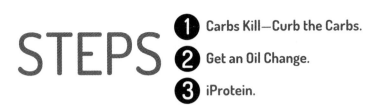

STEPS

1 Carbs Kill—Curb the Carbs.

2 Get an Oil Change.

3 iProtein.

1 Step 1. Carbs Kill—Curb the Carbs

Whether you eat a Snickers bar, an apple, or a bowl of rice, down the line the carbohydrates end up as sugar in your system. If all of this sugar energy is used, then it's not a problem. Additionally, some people are highly carb tolerant, and their body manages to absorb the excess energy they eat—at least for now.

The Quick Story on: Insulin

In the process of taking in sugar, the hormone insulin is required for the cells to absorb it. At modest doses of slow-burning sugars, this mechanism will serve you just fine and for a long, long time. It's excess energy that creates a problem.

That's where the problem in our nutritional story begins. The average person eats enough carbs every day to literally run the N.Y. Marathon –twice. Yet, many sit in front of a computer all day or at the very most, don't put in anywhere near that amount of activity mileage.

? But I Thought my Brain Needed Sugar?

One of the solutions we'll address to stop carbs from killing you is to make you more of a fat burner than a sugar burner. You may be thinking, "I thought you needed sugar for energy?" But that's not entirely true.

First, the body can synthesize its own glucose (a form of sugar) where needed. Second, by becoming a fat burner, you cause your body and brain to learn to rely on ketones called B-hydroxybutyrate and less sugar for fuel.

This is much better energy management and one of the core principles of Maximized Metabolix: When blood sugar is kept down, you switch to burning fats and making ketones, avoiding the many metabolic dangers of sugar.

Excess sugar requires excess insulin. If you're continually eating carbs, eventually the presence of insulin in the system gets ignored more and more by the cells. Too many carbs cause the insulin to keep knocking on the door of the cells (called "receptors"). But the cells start to ignore the knock, like we might ignore a bad neighbor. Insulin keeps calling and the cells just keep sending to voice-mail. This situation is called insulin resistance.

What's worse, the excess sugar then gets stored as fat, and other issues arise as the brain starts to become resistant to other fat and appetite-balancing hormones. In case that wasn't bad enough, this process also creates the inflammation and oxidation related to bad aging and worsening disease.

Another problem with excess sugar energy in the diet is that it can lead to excess triglycerides and create bad cholesterol. While these effects are generally blamed on fats, you'll find they're really more bad news about carbs.

In reality, getting fat is a metabolic marker of too much carb energy and the growing inability of your body to manage all the sugar and the excess fat it creates. Since the intake of more sugar than your body can manage causes obesity, obesity-related diseases, high triglycerides, bad cholesterol, and advanced aging, we say "carbs kill."

② Step 2. Get an Oil Change

When you restrict your carbs, you'll be getting more calories from fat. Fat is not "bad" as once thought. It's the right choice to make when choosing sources of energy.

> **Step 2** addresses the problem that most people's fatty acid balance is upside down and sideways.

Modern society has you getting the mass majority of your fats from omega-6s, eating too many trans fats, and getting very, very little omega-3s. As we'll cover, omega-6 is involved in creating inflammation, and omega-3 is anti-inflammatory.

It's also likely that you're eating a lot of commercially raised animal products which contain toxins and a poor, unbalanced assortment of fats.

Monounsaturated fats from whole foods like extra virgin olive oil and raw almonds are lacking in many diets. For some, there is an overemphasis on monounsaturated fats, which can be found in body fat, and an under-emphasis on MCTs (medium-chain triglycerides) from coconut oil that aren't found in body fat and even help you burn fat.

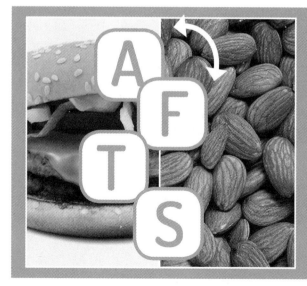

Fats out of Order

Too many people get their fats wrong. Some of the most frequent mistakes I see include:

- Too many omega-6s
- Too few omega-3s
- Too many commercial animal products
- Missing monounsaturated fats
- Missing MCTs
- Missing pasture-raised animal fats

You'll learn in this book that all types of fats, other than trans-fats, have benefits. It's just important to change the order of priority of your fats which also changes the amount of different fats in your diet. That's why we call this getting an "oil change."

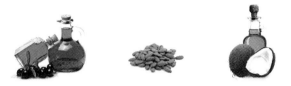

 ## Step 3. iProtein

Proteins (Greek: proteios, or "first," to imply the basis of life), are a huge and diverse class of organic compounds that are vital to every living cell. They are structural "building blocks," functional machinery, and can even be used as fuel.

Having regular protein in your diet is not only essential, but can help you lose fat, build and retain muscle, and keep athletic performance high as you go about the important work of reducing carb intake.

How much protein do you need? And how much can your body handle? As it turns out, the answers are highly individual.

That's why you need to stop thinking in terms of "protein" and start thinking in terms of what levels of protein are good for you: iProtein.

Another iProtein factor for meat and dairy eaters regards the kinds of protein you can get your hands on. Commercially fed and raised (non-organic) animal products have disturbed levels of fatty acids and are full of toxins, steroids, and antibiotics. In the chapter "iProtein," you'll learn more about good, whole sources of protein as well as the amounts of protein you'll need on a daily basis.

Age, weight, gender, activity level, and clean or unclean sources of animal products—these are all variables that impact your need for protein. We'll provide you the simple rules to make the right choices for you.

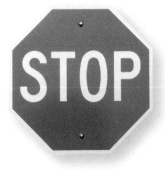

STARVING YOURSELF!

Here's some good news: if you want to lose weight, grow healthier, and increase longevity, you don't have to starve yourself. In fact, quite the opposite, you can eat a whole lot—as long as you're sticking to the formula.

H$_2$A$_2$ Eating:
Food and Physiology

 What happens to the food you eat once it enters your body?

That is the essential question of the Maximized Metabolix Formula. It asks you to probe deeper into the food you eat, not only viewing it as a storehouse of calories but as a storehouse of compounds, macronutrients, and substances that have varying effects on the complicated metabolic pathways of your body.

The formula considers the *physiology* of the food. It refers to what food does to your body after you eat it, rather than reducing all food to a simple caloric equation.

Let's break down food as simple caloric fuel vs. food and physiology— or what we call "Metabolix Foods."

Food as Fuel	Metabolix Foods
You are what you eat.	You are the impact food has on your body, including how that food is metabolized.
If I eat fat, I will get fat.	This is no truer than saying "if I eat vegetables, I'll become a vegetable." I'll show you how the body really increases fat stores and how to lose fat. Fat is the preferred fuel of the body and burns clean, without physiological harm.
Too much fat gives you heart disease.	Categorically wrong. Fats actually have benefits, and many fats, including saturated fats, have cardio-protective effects.
Cutting carbs = high protein	While your protein intake should be above survival guidelines, it shouldn't be "high."
It's my glands.	It might be. This is a diet based on hormones that get out of balance due to too much food energy.
I get vitamins and mineral from my diet.	Get the right amounts of vitamins and minerals needed to function—which almost always requires supplementation.
Carbohydrates are harmless energy, and as such, should be the staple of your diet. Whole grains, corn, and potatoes are healthy staples.	These "staples" raise blood sugar! In high quantities, they contribute to obesity, bad cholesterol, and diabetes.
Exercise more.	Exercise smart—it requires less time.
If it grows in the ground, it's healthy.	Well, broccoli grows in the ground—but so do potatoes and wheat. Poison ivy and worms grow in the ground also—but you don't eat them.
Eat less.	Eat more of the food that helps your physiology.

Throw Out Your Old Diet Books!

Whenever I speak to an audience, I ask three questions. First, I ask, "How many of you have at least two diet books in your house?" The whole room raises their hands and laughs.

Then, I ask, "How many of you have a whole weight-loss library?" More hands and laughing.

Finally, I inquire, "How many of you are currently still on any of those diets?" No hands or laughing—just some faint whimpers.

Yes, restricting almost any macronutrient in your diet can result in short-term weight loss. But what good is a diet if it ultimately results in a quick weight re-gain and no discernible long-term health benefits? A published 2007 review of calorie-restricted diet studies concluded, "there is little support for the notion that diets lead to lasting weight loss or health benefits."[2]

Traci Mann, an associate professor of psychology at UCLA and lead author of a calorie-restriction study, agreed, saying the majority of people in the study lost weight initially—but ultimately gained more weight than they lost, leading to no long-term health benefits.[3]

Are you depressed yet?

It's understandable. After all, we've been told for decades that the only way to lose weight was to practice discipline and fight our own hunger. If that was true, then the only "good food" is food that is lower in calories, no matter what other effect it has on our bodies once we begin digesting it. When we ultimately failed at our diets—as the science shows the majority of people do—we blamed ourselves and our lack of willpower. But what if willpower isn't the problem after all?

Food myth: You are what you eat

Truth: You are what your body is able to metabolically manage and what your system can make of it.

If it's processed and contains anything artificial or unnatural, but has the carbs, proteins, and or fats you're looking for – then it will still make you fat and sick. Many "health foods" aren't healthy.

If the old assumptions worked, we wouldn't be where we are today. It's time to throw out those old assumptions. I know, given what you've learned up until now about diets, it's hard to believe you can truly change how you eat without misery. But as Arthur C. Clarke once said, "Any sufficiently advanced technology is indistinguishable from magic."

That's what I want you to get out of this book: a sense that losing weight, gaining health, and earning more longevity is not only possible, it's not hard. In fact, it's "magically delicious."

The Tools to Conquer
the Diet Mountain

Kids will highlight the difficulty of getting people to consistently eat well. I have three kids. In their school, there's dessert anytime someone has a birthday. Some people bring muffins attempting to be "healthier," but a muffin is really just a cupcake eaten in the morning. (Look them up—they're really made of the same ingredients). Everyone knows you're not allowed to eat cake in the morning—unless it's cooked in a pan. Pancakes? Same ingredients - not sure how they snuck in there.

On the weekends, all of the kids have the actual birthday party. Here they are served sugar bread and frozen sugar milk. It's always eaten at the end so you'll take your kid home right away. No one wants to see what happens when thirty kids and a clown get together all hopped up on two thousand CCs of sugar.

I've found ice cream to be the "crack" of children. For a kid, it's obviously a physically addicting substance. If you're trying to eat healthier in your family, you can't even mention ice cream. I spelled ice cream in the car once to my wife. At the time my youngest son couldn't spell yet, but I forgot that my daughter could. She immediately said, "We're getting ice cream!" I said, "No, Daddy was just talking about ice cream." My daughter responded, "I want it now. I'll take strawberry."

I don't believe that anyone understands all of the challenges of eating well more than I do. Experiencing this battle myself all of my life and combining that with treating so many patients and helping people all of these years has really enlightened me about the obstacles people face in their everyday lives.

That is why we have loaded up this entire process with so many tools. There are recipes, meal plans, food lists, a carb counter, a protein counter, a supplement guide, and more. Additionally, since I've found it's important to have a coach, we train Maximized Living doctors and health providers and provide programs to teach, guide, and hold people accountable so they can conquer this dietary mountain, rather than fall victim to it like so many do.

CHAPTER ONE:

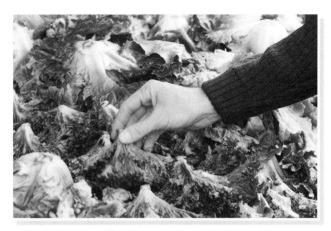

UPDATE YOUR NUTRITION

First, I want you to answer some very important questions.

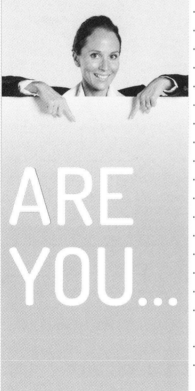

...a stress eater?
...a comfort eater?
...addicted to food or certain foods like sugar?
...in pain?
...suffering from severe arthritis?
...concerned about weight?
...low on energy?
...experiencing stomach trouble and/or digestive issues?
...dealing with high bad—or low good—cholesterol?
...demonstrating high triglycerides?
...experiencing Weight Loss Resistance (WLR)?
...having trouble with your hormones?
...suffering with an illness?
...struggling with depression, anxiety, or sleeplessness?
...worried about or struggling with the signs of aging?
...unsure what to feed your kids?
...unsure of what to eat because you're pregnant or thinking about having a child?
...overwhelmed with all of the supplement advice out there?
...a serious athlete or weekend warrior who wants to become better—or even the best?

If so, stay tuned—the information, foods, and eating plans you need are designed with you in mind.

"Eatin'," A Realistic Approach to Lifestyle Change

I had a bodybuilding friend in college who spent most of the day eating. One day, I asked him if he was hungry and wanted to go out to lunch. He said, "Hungry? What's that got to do with eatin'?"

Why do you eat? For some people, that sounds like a simple or maybe even a foolish question. They'd say, "For hunger or survival—right?" But people eat for a whole lot of different reasons.

People eat due to stress, for comfort, because they're addicted, because they're bored, for social reasons, because it's 6:00 p.m. and that's dinner time, and, occasionally, because a reduction in nutrients causes the brain to trigger certain hormones that indicate the need to feed on a particular type of food, a condition also known as actually being hungry.

I've eaten for all of the above reasons—and all in the same day. If you ask me, I'm with my old college buddy: for me hunger has little to do with "eatin'."

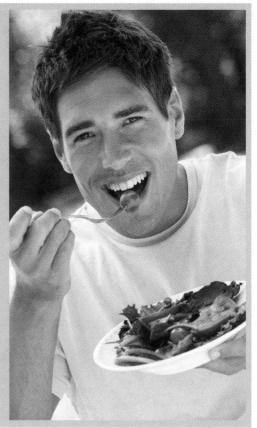

This is something not commonly addressed when people and programs reduce nutrition to a quick-fix diet. I'm not a psychologist and don't play one on television. As someone who got a degree in nutrition twenty-two years ago and who has worked with thousands of people trying to lose weight, I can tell you that most—if not all—dietary mind games and nutritional tricks don't work. It's just very tough to get past the different reasons why you decide to eat.

Rather than changing your mind about why you're eating, it's much easier to change what you're eating.

If you checked off any of the signs, symptoms, or the goals at the start of this chapter, the reasons why you eat become more costly. That's why we need methods that make lifestyle change more lasting. I eat when I'm bored. Frankly, that's just not changing. If I'm at my desk reading one scientific journal after another about the central nervous system or omega-3 fats, then I know I turn to food for comfort and sanity.

The key is, I know I can't be chowing down on carbs without paying the price.

The trick I've been sharing now for over a decade—with moms who are home all day with the kids, computer programmers, TV-watching snackers, truckers spending all day on the road, and those single men or women who just got dumped: you can eat for comfort with the right Metabolix foods.

Instead of cookies, pizza, or a half-gallon of Ben & Jerry's, what you'll find in front of our patients and on my desk at work are green apples, raw nuts, and our meal and dessert recipes. This method has worked for me now for decades.

A plan has to make your life easier, not harder than it is right now. You can't make it on a diet of deprivation. It just won't last. You want to be able to eat like an elephant, look like a gazelle, and still overcome your most common health concerns.

No-Guilt Chocolate Chip Cookies
(See? It's not all hopeless!)

Ingredients
- 2 1/2 cups almond flour
- 1/4 teaspoon sea salt
- 1/4 teaspoon baking soda
- 1/2–3/4 cup xylitol or if using stevia, add to taste
- 1 organic egg
- 1 tablespoon vanilla
- 1 stick (8 tablespoons) organic butter
- 1 bar sugarless chocolate, chopped into chunks

Directions
1. Preheat oven to 350 degrees.
2. Combine all the dry ingredients in a medium-sized bowl.
3. Melt the butter gently in a saucepan.
4. In a separate bowl, mix the butter with the egg and vanilla.
5. Add the wet ingredients to the dry ingredients and mix well.
6. Chop the chocolate bar and mix into the batter.
7. Drop tablespoons of batter an inch apart on a baking sheet.
8. Bake until slightly brown around the edges.

How to Gain Weight on Your Diet

I may have more compassion and understanding of people who struggle with their weight and their diet than anyone else on the planet. I've dealt with it literally all my life. My parents went on diet after diet. Even at seven or eight years old, I'd often diet with them. By the time I was eight, I could make a mean, fat-free, apple pie with a Grape Nuts crust, and I often ate Melba toast, celery, and cottage cheese for lunch in middle school.

No child should have to live through that.

The diet would always start on a Monday, and that decision always meant, "We'll never eat pizza, ice cream, Captain Crunch, or drink Coke, ever again!" On Sunday, we'd eat everything we knew we'd be deprived of for the rest of our lives.

Sadly, the diet would usually last only two–three days. As a matter of fact, sometimes the pressure would be too great, and the diet wouldn't start at all. All told, this would give us a net weight gain of approximately five–six pounds as a result of all of the food we ate on Sunday, before it started.

I was a personal trainer in my late teens; this is before we were even called "personal trainers." I was just that guy at the gym that helps you work out. At that time, nearly all of the people that approached me had the same goal: "I want to lose weight for—"spring break," "a trip to Hawaii," or "my wedding"—"which is coming up in two weeks."

Like you'd expect, this approach rarely worked. While some of them would really suck it up, work hard, and starve for those two weeks, they'd gain back every ounce and more immediately following their event. Like my parents' diets, in the end, the result from the start of the diet was weight gained, not lost. By the way, there's something not quite right about a man or woman dropping weight just for the wedding and then gaining more back.

That's like false advertising!

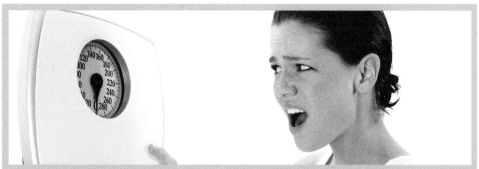

My experience with failing diets continued. In order to graduate with my degree in nutrition, I had to assist in a nutrition and weight-loss clinic. My first patient was a woman who was dating a friend of mine. She was beginning to put on a lot of weight, and she wanted to get it under control. Or, more likely, since he was the one who called, he wanted her to get it under control.

I gave her the standard diet program recommended by the nutritional science world at the time. It consisted of following a point scale. Each carbohydrate, protein, and fat gram was worth a certain number of points, and you were allowed only so many points per meal and per day. The object of this point system was to make sure you got the nutrients you needed while taking in only a certain amount of calories. One obvious problem with this method was that if you ate a cookie, that was it for food for the day.

Despite the fact that she handed in a diet diary every week showing that she was abiding by the system, every time she came in to see me, she had gained weight. At the end of her second week, she had gained eight pounds.

About that time, my friend called me and began to question what I was doing. In fact, he said, "You obviously have no idea what you are doing!"

With the painful reality that his girlfriend was packing on pounds at an alarming rate while under my care, and that the other clients I had started on the program also were gaining weight, I began to wonder if maybe he wasn't right.

The next day, as I pulled into the weight-loss clinic parking lot, I noticed my friend's girlfriend had arrived before me. I pulled up right next to her car to park, and as I got out of my car, I couldn't help but notice that her passenger seat was covered with colored sprinkles. As it turns out, part of her nutritionist appointment included a trip to Dairy Queen. This snack had not managed to make its way onto the weekly diet diary.

Great job, I thought to myself. As a result of your care, she now not only has an eating disorder, she's also become a pathological liar!

After watching all of my weight-loss patients gain an average of four pounds a week, and having all my diabetes patients end up doubling their insulin, it became clear that the standard methods of weight management the clinic was recommending weren't measuring up.

All of these diet plan failures sent me to the lab for the next several decades to find good science and plans that work. Now, I can look at a new fad diet or weight loss program and know in about four seconds whether or not it will work—or if it's so hard you'll just end up gaining more weight and smuggling ice cream products in your vehicle.

The Obesity Epidemic

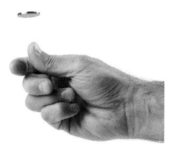

Do you have a quarter handy?
Good. I want you to flip it.

If you are an American adult, your chances of being overweight or obese are greater than the odds that you just flipped heads.[4] In fact, it's not even close. You have a fifty percent chance of flipping heads. But according to the latest statistics from the Center for Disease Control, there is an almost seventy percent chance that you are overweight or obese.

I was in an antique shop near my home in Central Florida and picked up a newspaper from the 1950s. Inside, was an advertisement for the circus that featured a picture of the "fat man." Immediately, I was struck by the fact that by contrast to the current public, he really didn't look that fat.

Today, the "fat man" of the 1950s would be a "medium" at Walmart.

As time goes by, the numbers are getting worse, not better. According to data from the National Health and Nutrition Examination Survey, obesity rates among children and adolescents have nearly tripled, with 12.5 million children aged 2-19 categorized as medically obese—the stage beyond merely "overweight." According to the Bogaluse Heart Study, children aged 5 to 17 are obese at a rate some three times the obesity rates in the early 1970s.[5]

Adults are no better off. The American Heart Association lists 154.7 million adults as overweight or obese. About one-third of all American adults are simply obese.[6]

In addition to costing us our health, obesity is costing us money. The CDC estimates the annual medical cost of obesity in the US was a staggering $147 billion in 2008 dollars, with obesity costing Americans an average of $1,429 more per year than people of average weight.[7]

That's a lot of quarters.

Switching to Carbs:
Getting Over the Wrong Ideas
of "Good Nutrition"

After a very incomplete record of scientific research, the so-called experts of the latter twentieth century made recommendations like, "Avoid fat and eat more carbohydrates."

And we listened.

For a generation, we were told that we should avoid fats—especially animal fats—if we wanted to be lean and healthy. But in order to replace those fat calories, we had to get our calories from somewhere else: grains, potatoes, corn, rice, and refined carbohydrates.

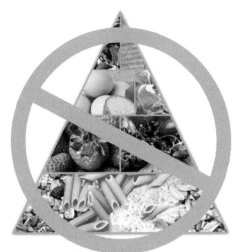

So we did. By 2000, the average American was consuming an average of 200 pounds of "flour and cereal products" per year, compared to 135 pounds in the early '70s. We listened to the Food Pyramid, too, increasing our grains from seven-and-a-half servings per day in the 1980s to ten servings per day in 2000.[8]

In 2013, the American Heart Association reported that Americans are eating more calories—and we're getting them from carbohydrates. "The increases in calories consumed … are attributable primarily to greater average carbohydrate intake, in particular, of starches, refined grains, and sugars."[9]

The question arises: If the simple "trick" was to eat less fat—particularly saturated fat—and less cholesterol, wouldn't most of us be leaner and healthier?

Yet obesity rates have never been so high, and its associated diseases have gone parabolic over the last fifty years. If the traditional definition of "good nutrition" is correct, and carbs are good, then how can this be?[10]

Metabolic Syndrome

Your weight and your diet are tied directly to your metabolic health. If you're overweight and not able to manage all of these carbs and other nutrients well, it's called "Metabolic Syndrome." Being overweight is correlated with a host of other diseases, from diabetes to cardiovascular disease. With the spread of Metabolic Syndrome, sometimes also called "Syndrome X," an increasing amount of Americans exhibits the following symptoms[11]:

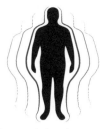

- **Poor body composition:** fatty weight is kept around the middle and upper parts of the body
- **High blood pressure:** Often higher than 130/85 mmHg
- **High cholesterol**
- **Inflammation**
- **High blood sugar:** a likely result of insulin resistance

If you exhibit these symptoms, you may have a higher risk of stroke, certain types of cancer, heart disease, kidney disease, diabetes, and even poor blood supply to the legs.

Diabetes

It's not a coincidence that, as our obesity rates skyrocket, the diabetes outbreak has come along for the ride.

After all, diabetes is a disease of metabolism. Type II diabetes means your body is not responding adequately to all of the insulin released by the pancreas to stabilize your blood sugar levels.

Suffering From Diabetes

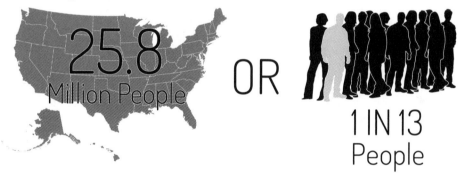

Today, some 25.8 million people in the United States suffer from diabetes, representing about one in every thirteen people. Of these, seven million people with diabetes don't even know they have it.

Combine this with some eighty million people suffering from prediabetes, and the numbers start to mirror the obesity epidemic.

Unsurprisingly, people who suffer from diabetes run many of the same risks as those with Metabolic Syndrome: high blood pressure, heart disease, stroke, kidney disease, along with other unpleasant side effects like neuropathic pain and even limb amputation.

According to the International Diabetes Federation, 350 million people suffer from this condition globally, a number which is expected to more than double by 2030.

It's well known that this is a condition not sparked by too much fat or just calories themselves, but all of the carbs.

"'Fats are Bad' and Other Hits," by Bill Haley and the Comets

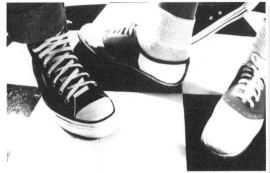

You can read more about how nutrition advice got skewed in the appendices. But for now, know that at the time of the study that started it all—the one claiming fats, particularly saturated fats, were bad—Bill Haley and the Comets were making songs to be played on an ancient musical device called a "record," and computers, with a fraction of the degree of complexity of your smart phone, took up 3100 square feet of space. There were no home computers at that time; the computers were a home.

When you start to look more closely at fat, you realize that the outdated advice to eat less fat makes no sense at all. Consider what we now know:

Fat Makes A Body Good

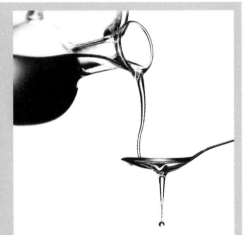

- There are several essential fatty acids that must be eaten to survive.
- The body needs fat to produce the steroid hormones testosterone, progesterone, and estrogen, which are based on cholesterol molecules.
- Fats slow the absorption of carbs, leading to normalized blood sugar.
- Dietary fats also give you the building blocks to build cell membranes (phospholipids).
- Fat is needed for vitamins A, D, E, and K to be absorbed and transported through the blood.
- Fats make up your brain tissue—we're all fatheads.
- Fats make up the lung surfactant, allowing you to breathe.
- Fats protect your organs.
- Some fats are anti-microbial and even body-fat burning.
- Fats are a body-preferred, clean source of energy.
- Saturated fat makes up a significant proportion of the most natural form of human food: breast milk.

You're probably saying, "But aren't saturated fats bad for you?"

Advice to replace saturated fat with unsaturated fat is unwarranted. No one has been able to show or prove mechanisms in the body that could show saturated fats to be "bad" and unsaturated fats to be "good." You can find the good, the great, and the bad in all types of fats, saturated and unsaturated alike.

Paradoxically, healthy human tissues continually make both saturated and unsaturated fats.

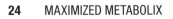

Saturated fats constitute half of the acids in cell membrane phospholipids and most of breast milk. There are many types of saturated fatty acids (SFAs) ranging in length from twelve to twenty-four carbons: three short, three medium, and three long chains. Are they all bad?

Well, your brain is made up of the long chain SFAs, arachidic and behenic. Your lung surfactant is made of the long chain palmitic acid. The medium chain lauric acid comprises a strong percent of breast milk and is antimicrobial (anti-fungal, ant-bacterial, and anti-protozoal).

Is that so "bad"?

Fat and Cholesterol:
Not So Simple as Once Thought

As nutrition science has matured, we now know that saturated fat, while it may or may not raise total cholesterol, also tends to raise good cholesterol. We're also discovering that the LDL that may be raised by saturated fats can often be the harmless kind of LDL.[12] We know for a fact that eating saturated fat doesn't necessarily mean you have greater amounts of saturated fat in your blood in the form of triglycerides. As you'll see later on, just the opposite is true.

Forty years ago, my dad was told he had high cholesterol. They didn't look at LDL or HDL numbers back then, so for all they really knew, the high cholesterol came from his good cholesterol. At any rate, he was told to avoid all foods that contained cholesterol.

By today's standards, this advice is downright moronic. We now know that cholesterol in the diet, except for extreme cases, does not raise serum cholesterol. The body is perfectly capable of balancing the cholesterol in the blood, whether or not we eat cholesterol in our diet. Yet, because he was told he had to avoid all of these rich, flavorful foods, my dad's life became miserable.

To read more about the history of diets, where the low-fat hypothesis came from, and how it's been proven to fail, see **Appendix II**.

Thomas Kuhn helped to father the meaning of the phrase "paradigm shift." He noted in his famous 1962 work, "The Structure of Scientific Revolutions," there are many traditions and complex sociological and economic factors that dispel logic and slow down or stop truth from entering into the mainstream.

Nutrition is an evolving science. You have to realize that yesterday's truth is today's misinformation. As the science improves, we're left to question some very old, traditional assumptions, many of which have turned out to be little more than myths.

As mentioned, while many continue to focus on calories as the main driver for nutrition, common sense and modern science dictate that one hundred olive-oil calories impacts your weight very differently than one hundred Hershey-bar calories.

The Prize

In the movie Jerry Maguire, Jerry called himself the "Lord of the Living Room." They'd send him in to a house to close a family with a young athlete on making him their agent. He had quite the pitch. On one call he said, "I will not rest until I have you holding a Coke, wearing your own shoe, playing a Sega game featuring you, while singing your own song in a new commercial starring you, broadcast during the Super Bowl, in a game that you are winning, and I will not sleep until that happens."

I researched and wrote the book with this in mind: I will not rest until I have you holding a smoothie, wearing a bikini or Speedo, while walking down the beach, showing off your body, which just got great reviews on Facebook, after you were just told your blood tests are perfect, getting ready to start a triathlon, and setting your PR (Personal Record).

KEY CONCEPTS FROM THIS CHAPTER

1. "Low fat" and "low calorie" diets don't work.

The nation was told to avoid fat in the latter half of the twentieth century, and where has it gotten us? We're more obese and diabetic than ever before. It's not a coincidence. Low fat and low calorie diets don't work because they ignore the principles of whole food and physiology you'll learn while reading this book.

2. The "fat = disease" myth is just that: a myth.

In this book, you'll learn how to eat the right fats in the right quantities to ensure a healthy waistline and a body free of inflammation. You won't be fed the myth that any and all fats will give you heart disease; in fact, you'll learn that today's science says that just about the opposite is often the case.

3. You aren't what you eat; you're what you do with what you eat.

When you eat sugar, you **don't** become sugar. When you eat bread, you **don't** become bread. It's also true that when you eat fat, you **don't** automatically become fat. It's not about what you eat so much as it is about the metabolic effects your food has on your body. Your body metabolizes, digests, and absorbs different nutrients through an entire "highway system" of effects. Eating right means knowing that "you are what you eat" is nothing more than a myth.

CHAPTER TWO:

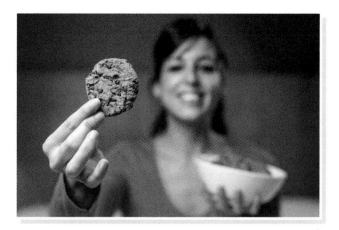

How Food Makes You Fat
Why You Gain Weight:
It's All About Your Hormones

Early on in my nutrition career, many of my overweight patients would come to me and say, "It's my glands."

To which I'd think, Sure—your salivary glands. (I wouldn't say it out loud, of course.)

For the most part, people are not victims of some kind of glandular foul play. Yet modern lifestyle and nutrition really have downloaded a serious gland virus and thus thrown off the effectiveness of our hormones to control metabolism and weight. So much so, you may need to reboot your hormones.

Hormones regulate virtually every aspect of your body's metabolic pathways and do it in very diverse ways. They cause you to either store or burn fat and build or tear down muscle. They make you feel full or hungry, and they handle about a million other functions that factor into your weight, fitness, and overall well-being.

Ultimately, hormones determine why you gain weight.

Hormones determine whether you're the kind of person who can eat cookies and pizza every day and stay skinny (the people we hate), or if you just simply walk by a bakery and put on twenty-five pounds.

The goal of any solid, weight loss plan has to address your glands. That's why we call our plans "diets based on hormones," or "hormonally-based eating." This is important to not just lose or maintain your weight, but to up the lean muscle and decrease the body fat. If you're lighter and not leaner, you're not necessarily healthier. You'll just die lighter. As a married man, who is father to a teenage boy, a pre-teen girl, and a six-year-old that is all boy, I can tell you that of all the differences between you and a machine, hormones are probably the greatest. It's not just what you eat, it's how food affects your hormones that matters most. If it's not a diet based on hormones, it's really not a diet.

Metabolix Weight Loss:
You Aren't What You Eat, You Are
What You Do With What You Eat

"You are what you eat" simply doesn't apply anymore. Your body's relationship with food is far more complex than this, which is really why "carbs kill" and Step 1 to the H_2A_2 formula will be such a consistent theme in this section.

What you eat will have a lot to say about your physical and mental destiny. Even if eating a plate of grapes doesn't turn you purple and round like Violet Beauregarde in *Willy Wonka*, remember that your body is more sophisticated than a simple closed system of one gas tank and one engine.

If you are what you eat, then you would have to believe that olive oil is more fattening than carbs because olive oil has nine calories/serving and carbs and proteins have only four. Yet olive oil and pasta do completely different things to your body.

Because of the hormonal impact carbs have on your body versus the hormonal impact of fat, you're far more likely to get fat on the carbs then fat on the fat.

The Hormones That Control Weight
and Body Composition:

Insulin

When broken down, carbohydrates are quickly released into the bloodstream, raising blood sugar. Your body must counteract the rise in blood sugar and bring it back to a healthy level. That's insulin's job.

The Role of Insulin in Managing Blood Sugar

Insulin encourages sugar (glucose) absorption by the muscles and slows down or stops the liver from releasing more, stored sugar (glycogen).

In a heavily carb-based diet, insulin stays chronically high for most people—unless you are an incredible carb burner. Eventually, the receptors on the cells become resistant to insulin.

insulating device preventing conductors.

insulin /'msjolin/ *n.* produced in the pan which regulates the the lack of which ca

If insulin cannot do its job, you are "insulin resistant." You are essentially allergic to carbs and metabolically compromised. As a result, the rise in blood sugar cannot be effectively assimilated into the cells.

The cells suffer insulin burnout and won't let the sugar in. At this point, among other things, the excess sugar is made into and stored as fat.

This opens up Pandora's box and lets out hormone madness.

Leptin

While a resistance to insulin alone can cause weight gain, it also impacts other fat- and weight-management hormones. One of these is leptin.

If insulin is the "fat hormone," then leptin is the "fat manager."

Leptin

Leptin works in the hypothalamus, stimulating metabolism and inhibiting appetite through a number of mechanisms.

Leptin works as an "energy balance indicator." Leptin levels circulate in the blood in correspondence to levels of body fat.

Some of the roles of leptin in metabolism include:
- inhibiting appetite by countering neuropeptide Y and anandamide. Both are feeding stimulants;
- inhibiting appetite by stimulating melanocyte-stimulating hormone α-MSH, which suppresses appetite and effects other body functions;
- helping control energy expenditure.

Health Comments

A review in *Nature* found that "human obesity is generally associated with an insensitivity to leptin."[13]

Leptin is your energy balance hormone. It helps regulate your appetite (and thus the energy you take in) and stimulates your metabolism. Leptin comes from body fat. The more body fat you have, the more leptin you'll see circulating in the bloodstream. When levels are high, it tells your brain that it has enough fat energy to burn and to stop eating.

More leptin isn't better! If there's insulin resistance, you're storing too much fat. As with too much insulin, too much fat causes the brain to start ignoring leptin, and the body keeps producing more. Leptin keeps calling, but the brain just lets it go to voicemail. You then become "leptin resistant"—a state in which the body is telling the brain to shut down hunger and burn fat, but the brain isn't listening.

Ghrelin

When you feel hungry, it's not simply because your stomach is empty. Ghrelin is one of the reasons an empty stomach is so often associated with hunger, serving as a link between your gut and your brain.

Source in the Body:

Ghrelin has been labeled a "stomach hormone," in the scientific literature[14], but evidence suggests it is produced in other places, such as pancreatic cells, as well.

Ghrelin

The "hunger hormone."

Levels rise with lack of sleep, and balance is affected by body weight.

Ghrelin is partially to blame for your hunger—and your subsequent desire to eat fattening junk food to satisfy it. When it comes to being able to make the right call at a restaurant and choose the chicken or the fish rather than the pizza or fettuccine Alfredo, some of it will have to do with this hormone. The rest will have to do with how much you enjoy having working arteries.

When you're lacking sleep, or if you're overweight, ghrelin is raised, leading to even more hunger and adding an additional obstacle in your goal to be fit.[15]

The Hormone Cascade

Once insulin is off, as we've discussed, it sets off a cascade of different hormone effects.

Here's How it Works:

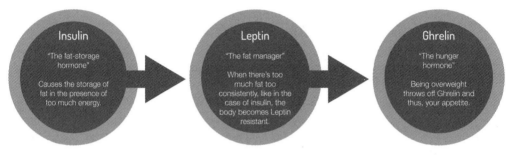

As you can see, this is one example of how hormones can have a negative domino effect in the body.

If you have insulin and leptin resistance, along with ghrelin malfunction, you're seriously hormonal. It's like Flounder getting chastised by Dean Wermer in *Animal House*, when he says, "Fat, drunk, and stupid is no way to go through life, son."

Fat, maybe. But stupid and drunk? All three is way too much.

Yes, like many people, once you're insulin- and leptin-resistant and other weight managers like ghrelin get out of line, you've got issues. Yet, there is good news. If you get insulin sensitivity under control, you'll lose weight—and fat and these hormones will move back in the right direction.

The eating plans you'll discover in the upcoming chapters address these hormones. Specifically, they address your carb tolerance, which has shown over and over to get insulin under control and reverse a very real, negative hormone cascade. *(See the carb section, Chapter 4, to determine your carb tolerance.)*

Curb Carbs, Curb Hunger

Findings show that a high-protein breakfast decreased the presence of ghrelin "more strongly over time" than did a high-carbohydrate breakfast.[343]

You can turn this around by curbing the carbs. Following Maximized Metabolix eating strategies for weight loss, cutting carbs, and/or increasing the fats in your diet will push insulin, leptin, ghrelin, testosterone, and cortisol toward more desirable levels.[16, 17, 18, 19, 20, 21]

Other Hormones to Address

- Testosterone, a muscle-making hormone that exists in both genders and helps preserve lean tissue, which makes it something of an "anti-cortisol."
- Cortisol, the so-called, "stress hormone," that can lead to muscle tissue loss. Some studies also indicate that a low-fat diet can trigger chronically high levels of cortisol.

Mixed Sweet Nut Recipe

Ingredients
- 5 cups of raw, whole almonds and/or pecans
- 1 egg white
- 1 tablespoon of water
- Beat with nuts
- Mix with 1/2 cup xylitol
- 1 tablespoon cinnamon
- Pinch of salt

Directions
1. Mix together
2. Cook for 15 min. at 350 degrees
3. Stir and cook for another 10–15 min. until browned.

*See the weight-loss appendix, **Appendix IV**, for more on dealing with testosterone and cortisol.*

The good news? The H_2A_2 formula and nutrition plans will handle most of the hormone changes needed. But, as we'll cover here, sometimes, you'll need to do more.

Addressing Weight Loss Resistance (WLR)

Many people will shift their food to natural, whole sources and BAM, they see instant changes. Others, whose hormones are more shot, will need to address carb intolerances and observe the plans more closely to see similar results. The degree of your hormonal imbalance will determine how simple or involved keeping or getting weight off will be. My very first weight-loss discovery was this: Just by eating whole, natural food, you would drop weight. You could eat your weight in fruits and vegetables and usually lose weight.

I once helped a family of eight switch from processed to natural foods. It led them not only to achieve their desired weight without being hungry, but they were able to shed many of their medical problems like asthma, allergies, ear infections, and chronic colds and flues. This family of eight helped me write my first recipe book after this all-important shift.

The people who lose weight quickly on this plan often do so because they address their metabolic dysfunction in the earlier stages of the diet. If their hormones are generally healthy, it won't be hard for them to make the shift (All they need is what is the Core Plan). I've seen some people cut out sodas and fast food and immediately drop thirty pounds.

For many, however, factors including the modernization of food, stress, a sedentary lifestyle, and/or the endless toxins that have infiltrated our food and personal care products have created much physiological damage and made them very resistant to losing weight. In these cases, just cutting back on Sprite won't quite do the trick (they need the Advanced Plan).

More on Weight Loss Resistance

Most people will see great results taking the dietary steps we'll walk you through in the next few chapters. For others, it may not be quite so easy. In their case, due to more extreme metabolic damage, they'll need to heed some additional nutritional tips and to address other lifestyle issues to get back on track.

Here are the other areas of WLR you may need to address:
- Testosterone
- Cortisol
- Toxins
- Stress and sleep (which affect hormones)
- Intensity and duration of exercise
- Gluten, fructose, and triglycerides

*Check out **Appendix IV** for tips on how to address each of those problems.*

KEY CONCEPTS FROM THIS CHAPTER

1. Eat to correct your hormones.

Most of the diet advice out there is centered on counting calories, tracking portion sizes, and trimming the fat. None of that advice focuses on correcting your body's hormonal environment. If you eat Metabolix, you'll be well on your way to correcting the negative "hormone cascade" that results from too much carb energy.

2. You may need to address Weight Loss Resistance.

As you may well be aware, some people go on diets and seem to correct their metabolic problems overnight. Other people are not so lucky. If you're one of the unlucky ones, you may need to correct your WLR, or Weight Loss Resistance. *You can find more on Weight Loss Resistance in Appendix IV.*

CHAPTER THREE:

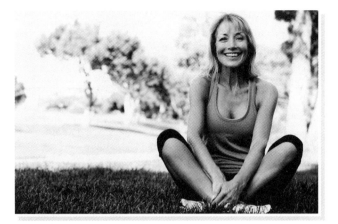

HOW DIET MAKES YOU AGE

Is Fifty the New Twenty?

Years ago, someone started the trend that "Forty is the new thirty." That's actually not entirely true. Really, fifty is the new thirty—or maybe even the new twenty.

Yet, the unfortunate tendency is to go quietly into that good night—and not put up a fight. There's actually a theory on aging that says it's all in your belief system. The theory is that it all starts when you're a child. You see a man bent over and going by on a walker and you ask your parents, "Why is that man walking like that?"
You parents say, "Because he's old."
"How old," you say.
"Seventy or eighty," they respond.

To which you immediately think to yourself, So that's how I'll be at seventy or eighty. Got it. Don't get caught up believing that old age is creeping up on you. I see this happen with patients and many people I know. As they age, they start expecting to slow down. I see some folks as early as in their twenties and early thirties believing that the knee pains that stop them from exercising—or their back pain and sleeping troubles—are "normal" signs of aging, what to expect from what they've experienced or done to themselves in the past.
It's all a big, fat, hairy lie.

The truth is, with what we know today about the Five Essentials of Maximized Living (in this case the Nutrition Essential), aging doesn't have to mean getting old. We've seen tens of thousands of occasions when people who believed they were stuck with a condition of old age merely needed to change their diet.

So many of the patients we've dealt with on their low-fat high-carb diets had stopped exercising and doing many of the activities they did when they were "younger" because of "my knee" or "my feet," etc. Now, as long as they eat the way we're going to show you here, they can play sports with the kids again, workout, sleep, go running, or—at the very least—have run out of excuses.

Personally, I tried the Disney Marathon when I was twenty-nine. It was an ugly, painful, epic journey that I believed permanently ended my running career. I finished in a slow five hours, dragging my right leg out of sheer force of will for the last ten miles. A patient who saw me at mile seventeen said, "Dr. Ben, you didn't look so good."

"Kitchen Sink" Yogurt

Ingredients

- Organic, plain, whole or goat's milk yogurt—if your are dairy sensitive
- Shaved, unsweetened chocolate
- Stevia, to taste
- 1 cup raspberries, blueberries, strawberries, or combo 1/4 cup ground flax seed and/or chia seeds

Optional:

- Shredded coconut
- 1 teaspoon almond or peanut butter

Directions

1. Combine ingredients into blender.
2. Blend to desired consistency.

Thankfully, I made the diet switch. Now, instead of a painful five hours, I comfortably run a marathon in the low threes at the age of forty-seven. So maybe fifty is the new twenty.

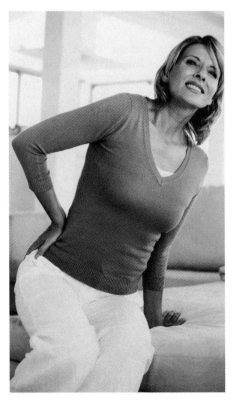

Inflammation and Oxidation
The Markers of Aging and Chronic Disease

Inflammation

Acute inflammation is a healthy part of your body's defense system. You need it to manage injury, infection, and the healing process. On the other hand, excess, long-term, or chronic inflammation is a major cause of disease in the modern world.

Modern health science pays careful attention to signs that your body is in an inflammatory state. There are key mediators, or "biomarkers," that you can find in the blood that accurately measure how well you're aging and whether or not you're developing the common diseases of the elderly.

Inflammation is not only linked to cancer and heart disease, but diabetes, arthritis, hypertension, autoimmune disease, and aging, itself.

These markers of inflammation and pro-inflammatory cytokines that can be found in your blood, such as:

Inflammation Markers in your Blood
Tumor necrosis factor-alpha (TNF-alpha)
C-reactive protein (CRP)
Interleukin-6 (IL-6)

really tell you a whole lot about your present and your future.

You may not know that the presence of markers like CRP put you at many times the risk of a heart attack than the presence of LDL cholesterol.[22]

The good news is that these measures are tightly tied to lifestyle and therefore well within your power to control.

Oxidation

Another factor in health and aging with a strong nutritional component is oxidation or oxidative stress.

The number one nutrient keeping you alive isn't Starbucks—or even an apple. It's oxygen. You're surrounded by it, you breathe it, and you're energized by it. As your body continually interacts with oxygen, this causes oxidation or oxidative stress.

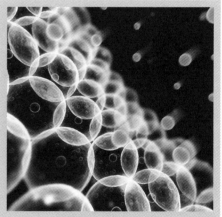

The damaging part of oxidative stress is the production of what's called ROS, or "reactive oxygen species," more commonly known as "free radicals."

Your body is designed to naturally respond to oxidation through anti-oxidation (anti-oxidants). Free radicals can cause damage to all of the components of your cells, down to the DNA. If your anti-oxidants can't keep up, you're more prone to a list of diseases, more inflammation,[23] and you speed up the aging process.

Toxins, emotional stress, radiation, physical stressors like intense exercise, sugar, weight gain, insulin issues, inflammation, and glycation (discussed later in this chapter) can increase oxidation and make it even more difficult for your antioxidant defenses to keep up. So you can see where inflammation and oxidation are closely tied in terms of cause and impact.[24]

The Dietary Causes of Old Age
Spoiler Alert: It's Carbs Again.

Unhappy aging and chronic disease have far more to do with nutrition and other important living essentials than the fact that someone is simply getting older. Anti-aging health practices are not about stopping the clock. It's not the clock's fault. They're about slowing inflammation, oxidation, and other related factors mentioned here. It starts with the knowledge that carbs help make you old. Taking in carbs and sugar generates inflammation and increases free radicals.[25, 26] This worsens as you develop the conditions of excess carb energy intake, i.e., your body becomes overweight, insulin resistant, and/or you begin living in a pre- or current state of type 2 diabetes.[27, 28]

As it turns out, science has already established a number of ways you can reduce and even reverse chronic inflammation by examining some of the most common causes of bodily stressors.

The answer isn't anti-inflammatory drugs. Using medications to shut down the mechanisms of inflammation, rather than addressing the causes of inflammation, is masking the symptom. This lets the causes continue to wreak havoc on your body, causing unpleasant side-effects.

While there are several other lifestyle factors involved here, the first place to look is your diet. The good news is that as you restrict glucose-producing foods and lose weight, there is a direct correlation with better insulin sensitivity, less inflammation, less free-radical exposure, and radically improved prospects for your heart and overall health.

In reducing chronic inflammation and oxidation, it's important to know that they're consistently caused by a few dietary culprits, and they're consequent metabolic impact. Let's look at the main culprits.

The Forces of Aging
Three Culprits that Ignite the Inflammatory, Free-Radical Fire

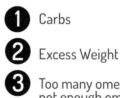

1 Carbs

2 Excess Weight

3 Too many omega-6s and not enough omega-3s

1 Carbs

They kill and they age. Carbs trigger insulin to a far greater degree than proteins—and fats don't trigger it at all. The presence of insulin kicks in many inflammatory biomarkers. As you'll see in the following table, the presence of insulin is strongly associated with inflammation.

The Facts Behind Sugar, Insulin, and Inflammation

Conclusions	Where Published?
Biomarkers for inflammation like C-reactive protein and interleukin 6 were predictive of developing type-2 diabetes.	**Journal of the American Medical Association, 2001**[29]
All sorts of markers for inflammation, including TNF-alpha, IL-6, IL-8, MCP-1, etc., were improved under a very low-carb diets. Quite simply, the subjects eating fewer carbs and more fat saw inflammation improve.	**Lipids, 2008**[30]
Link between high sugar, high glycemic-index foods, and inflammatory diseases.	**American Journal of Clinical Nutrition, 2010**[31]
A link between insulin and the inflammatory marker C-reactive protein.	**Journal of Clinical Hypertension, 2010**[32]

But there's more to the story of why carbs kill than just insulin. You also have to factor in AGEs.

Carbs and AGEs
Advanced Glycation End-Products

If you live long enough, eventually you're going to die.

While the statistics on aging are still that it affects one out of one, if you want to slow it down, look into the issue of advanced glycation end-products or AGEs. The acronym AGE is appropriate, because that's what AGEs give you: more aging.

What are they? They're the result of blood glucose going up and reacting with protein to form a glucose-protein molecule.

This is yet another reason sugar is not your friend! Sugar creates AGEs—whether it's from eating straight-up white sugar, from natural sweeteners like honey and maple syrup, or from whole or refined grains. The end-products created by any of these carbs, or AGEs, have a hand in aging by making your body's cells stiffer and less responsive. AGEs travel throughout the body and are connected to kidney disease, atherosclerosis, dementia, cancer, erectile dysfunction, eye disease, and other conditions.

How AGEs Cause Problems in Your Body

These AGEs will accumulate in blood vessel walls, where they affect the structure and even the function of your body's cells.[33] In the presence of diabetes, it has even been "implicated," as one American Heart Association study put it, as a major reason diabetics suffer from so many vascular complications.

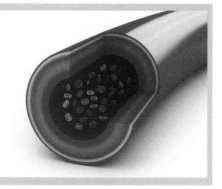

In addition to aging tissue, AGEs cause oxidation and inflammation.[34, 35]

While AGEs still form when blood sugar levels are normal, it's at a much lower rate. The higher your blood sugar is, the more AGEs you make. The good news, once again, is, as with the other causes of inflammation, disease, and aging, you can reduce AGEs by reducing or avoiding sugar in your diet. A 2001 study found that since vegetarians tend to have a diet higher in fructose and glucose, they had a higher amount of AGEs in their blood than did omnivores.[36, 37] While it's true you can eat AGEs in your diet through many protein-rich foods, it's unlikely they end up causing harm in your system.[38] As in the case of saturated fat, eating something does not mean that it will necessarily raise that same substance in your blood levels. If you want to avoid AGEs, the Fountain-of-Youth solution should sound familiar: Curb the carbs.

NOTE: We're not eliminating carbs altogether. Each of us has a certain carb tolerance. This will improve as you get your diet under control. As you've seen, your tolerance goes beyond just your weight: it can tell your future.

Excess weight

Simply being overweight spurs inflammation. The pro-inflammatory cytokines we've been discussing, like TNF-alpha, are closely related to adipose tissue, or body fat, and are, by extension, related to metabolic problems.[39]

CRP, another major inflammatory marker, increases with the condition of overweight.

Too many omega-6s and not enough omega-3s

In the chapter on fat, we'll establish that omega-3s decrease inflammatory substances (like proinflammatory cytokines)[40]. These have been called, "potent anti-inflammatory agents." Omega-6s on the other hand are inflammatory.

You'll see how by keeping your relative levels of omega-6s to omega-3s healthy through lowering the 6s and adding the 3s, you'll have taken another major step in solving inflammation and its related conditions.

It's Never Too Late to Fight Aging

By following the Five Essentials of Maximized Living, people are taking an aggressive stance against disease or recovering from even advanced stages of illness. Over the years, we've had so many people with very severe cases walking into our clinics. Years ago, I had an elderly woman carried in to my office by her family. It turns out this poor woman had been sent home to hospice to die. She was very ill and hadn't moved in over a decade.

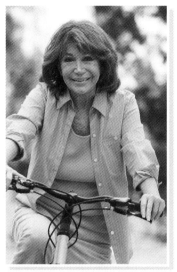

After starting her on the plan, I really felt like if we were going to win against all odds, she had to get moving. We came up with a strategy to prop her up on a stationary bike at home and, if necessary, her family could physically help her legs move against the pedals, just to get her going.

A couple of weeks later—weeks we weren't even sure we'd have when we started—the family came in very excited. They said, "She's doing five now!"

I responded, "Great—five minutes is awesome!" To which they said, "No, five rotations."

The miracle was that by continuing to eat the Maximized Metabolix way and follow these Essentials, she eventually left hospice and was riding around her neighborhood on a real bike.

She got young again. It's really never too late.

A Quick Guide to Cholesterol

Most people are taught that cholesterol is the virtual "monster in the bedroom" for people over thirty. It hides out under the bed—or, in this case the blood stream—ready to pop up and kill you.

On the contrary, cholesterol isn't your enemy. It does many important, good things in your body.

We need cholesterol. Cholesterol is a vital component in forming and healing all membranes in all animal cells. So without cholesterol, there is no "us."

Cholesterol is a perfectly natural, biological molecule. It's meant to help your body. Your body uses cholesterol as a "raw material" to make many hormones, like vitamin D and steroid hormones.

Dietary cholesterol—or the cholesterol we eat from animal products like eggs—is readily absorbed into the gut. But cholesterol is also produced by our body, usually in the liver. Dietary cholesterol does not control cholesterol levels in your blood. The body balances hormone levels. If you eat more cholesterol, you make less. If you eat less, you make more.

The understanding of cholesterol is still evolving. I speak to many of the labs around the US that study this important body substance. The traditional understanding and advice surrounding cholesterol has become outdated.

Types of Cholesterol	
High-density lipoproteins (HDL), or "HDL cholesterol."	Commonly known as the "good" cholesterol, these lipoproteins transport cholesterol to the liver rather than to artery walls. As a scavenger of excess cholesterol from lipoproteins and tissues, these can actually help prevent heart disease. *What is not commonly known:* there are multiple types of HDLs. The smaller, less mature ones are not as healthy as the larger versions.
Low-density lipoproteins (LDL), or "LDL cholesterol."	Commonly known as the "bad" cholesterol. These carry cholesterol from the liver to the cells and the arteries that require it. Like HDL, new findings show us that there are different types of LDL particles. Understanding the difference can be very important in reading your cholesterol panel: • VLDL or "very low-density lipoprotein," which carries triglycerides and is a precursor to LDL particles. • LDL-A are large and fluffy, and generally regarded as harmless. • LDL-B are smaller, harder, and denser, and can promote atherosclerosis.

While the idea was once that you get more fat and cholesterol in the blood from eating fat and cholesterol, the science has come to show this is not the case.

Actually, it's more likely that too many carbs will cause the excess sugar to be converted to fat by the liver. As fat has to be carried through the blood as cholesterol, this forces cholesterol to go up. This is actually how you produce the more dangerous cholesterol and lipid profile that causes cardiovascular disease.

The Other Lipoprotein

Apoliproteins, inflammation, and oxidation

Apolipoprotein A (LP(a)), in a healthy system, repairs damage to blood vessels. However, in the event of too much inflammation, it can form plaque and being thrombogenic, LP(a) can also promote the formation of clots in blood vessels.

Apolipoprotein B has great susceptibility to oxidative damage by free radicals, more easily penetrate arterial walls, stay in circulation longer, and contribute to atherosclerosis.

After the sugar is converted to fat in the liver, the body then kicks out triglyceride carrying chylomicron and triglycerides. High triglycerides are a major risk factor for death.

Additionally, these triglycerides get packed into the VLDLs. VLDLs are the upstream precursor to immature, small, dangerous atherosclerotic LDL particles.

Carbs and Cholesterol:
A Bigger Link Than You Think

Most people would say (since typical carbs like rice, potatoes, and pasta are "cholesterol free") that it's the fat that raises the cholesterol.

Glucose in the blood can be converted to both fatty acids and cholesterol, which is why carbohydrates can have a cholesterol-raising effect. We were told to avoid fat and eat carbohydrates instead, but this was really good marketing and not good science.[41]

Addressing Cholesterol with Food

Another problem with excess energy in the diet is that it can create cholesterol directly. This is the metabolic pathway that statin "cholesterol" drugs inhibit. Obviously it would be better to address the excess energy issue than to try to stop it with a dangerous drug designed to shut down physiologic mechanisms in the body.

The reason all drugs have "side-effects" is that they're designed to shut something down. This is never a great choice if you can avoid it. The main cause of dangerous gains in fat and bad cholesterol is too much sugar and not too much fat. Better to address that, as suggested in the chapters to come, then to look to medications.

Raise Your Cholesterol IQ

If you want to sound really smart at a party, tell people it's not high cholesterol that's the problem and lowering cholesterol with drugs like Lipitor isn't the life-saving solution. When oxidation and inflammation meet those cholesterol particles, it's like Adele's song, "I set fire to the rain" – they make the cholesterol a dangerous foe to be reckoned with. Controlling these two major elements of aging are real solutions to the normal and necessary process of circulating cholesterol.

Key Concepts From This Chapter

1. Aging is not only about time.

"Premature" aging is caused by chronic inflammation, oxidation, and other biomarkers for bodily stress we've been talking about throughout this chapter. They say that "Age ain't nothin' but a number," and it's true—but only if you take proactive steps to curb carbs and improve the quality of your fat and protein sources. You'll learn more about accomplishing exactly that in the coming chapters.

2. Carbs shift cholesterol balance and size in the wrong direction and raise unwanted triglyceride levels.

By curbing the carbs and raising the fats—as we've been discussing—you're likely to shift your cholesterol numbers away from the small, more dangerous particles and towards the larger, less harmful particles. You'll also lower your triglyceride levels.

THE METABOLIX FORMULA:

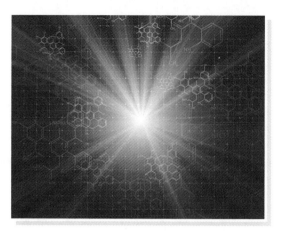

H_2A_2
A Formula for Change

As you're beginning to see, the issues you and everyone else are facing today keep coming back to curbing carbs and taking the right approach to the foods that are left—protein and fats.

Like the chemical formula for water is H_2O, the Maximized Metabolix formula for life is H_2A_2. While most diet programs only focus on weight, we also want to keep you alive— so this very effective formula addresses the causes of weight gain, disease, and aging, like hormones, inflammation, oxidation, and AGES that we've been covering.

As you'll recall, H_2A_2 stands for:
- (H_2) Happy Hormones, Healthy Weight Loss
- (A_1) Anti-inflammatory
- (A_2) Anti-aging

There are Three Steps to this formula:

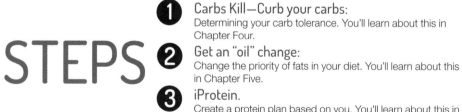

STEPS

1 Carbs Kill—Curb your carbs:
Determining your carb tolerance. You'll learn about this in Chapter Four.

2 Get an "oil" change:
Change the priority of fats in your diet. You'll learn about this in Chapter Five.

3 iProtein.
Create a protein plan based on you. You'll learn about this in Chapter Six.

The goal of our doctors is to always to make people's lives easier. So you'll find that the components of the formula in the next four chapters are all embedded in two plans, the Core and Advanced Plans. You can also take the Life Risk Questionnaire at the beginning of the Appendices to find out which plan and course of action is best for you.

Next, we'll move through the carbs, fats, and proteins you'll eat to address these three steps and put the Metabolix Formula to work.

CHAPTER FOUR:

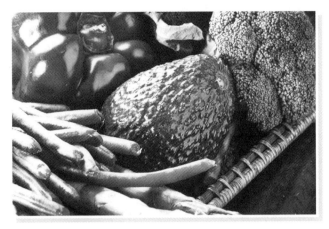

Carbs Kill:
Curb the Carbs

H₂A₂ Formula Step 1

As you've seen, carbohydrates are a big part of the cause of weight gain, aging, and poor health. Curb the carbs to correct the cause.

While the need for this step is pretty clear, I realize from the popularity of candy and the stock price of Coca-Cola, Inc., that for some, curbing carbs is no easy task.

I'll supply you with all of the tools to make the necessary improvements: the good carbs lists, meal plans and recipes, the Carb Counter, and plenty of allowable desserts (in **Chapter Eight**).

Examples of Good Carbohydrates for Your Kitchen	
Best Foods (Advanced Plan)	• High fiber vegetables (Examples: asparagus, broccoli, cabbage, Brussels sprouts, kale, cauliflower, and lettuce) • Avocados • Berries and Granny Smith apples • Granola/dry cereal—gluten-free, sugar-free, no chemicals or trans-fats *(See our recipe section to learn how to make your own.)* • Coconut milk and flour
Foods in Moderation (Advanced Plan)	• Beans and lentils *(See our "soaked and sprouted" section in Appendix IX for preparing these.)* • Raw cashews, filberts, pecans, and almonds *(Soaking helps make these more digestible.)*
Foods for the Active, Carb-tolerant, and Young (Core Plan)	Whole grain, organic, gluten-free snacks that don't use potato, white rice, corn, or starches. **Many imposters here!** • Oats, oatmeal (gluten-free is best.) • Dried fruit without sulfites or added sugars • Raw, organic honey • Coconut water for recovery of multi-hour exercise • Gluten-free ancient grains: amaranth, quinoa, millet, buckwheat • Brown rice

(More lists to come)

"Bender's Proverb"

I live near Disney World. I'm assuming due to the mega availability of junk food, the theme parks here in Orlando draw throngs of people that have very serious weight issues. Because of my family's history with obesity and the devastating effects it's had on us, my heart breaks when I look at these "Magic Kingdom" crowds.

But my biggest concern is that it's not just the weight. Lurking beneath the pounds is a serious hormone crisis that is leading to much pain, suffering, and deadly illness.

There's something I call "Bender's Proverb." In the movie The Breakfast Club, the character John Bender, played by Judd Nelson, calls Claire (Molly Ringwald) fat. When she objects, since she's not actually overweight, he says, "[You're] not fat at present, but I can see you really pushing maximum density. There are two kinds of fat people: there's fat people and there's fat people that were once thin but became fat."

Too many carbs mess with critical hormones. While you may appear to have it under control—or even be thin and lean—the carbs will kill you, over time. With the regular consumption of sugar and sugar-producing foods, your cells and tissues are becoming more and more desensitized to insulin and that makes fat! As fat builds up, your body also stops listening to fat-controlling hormones like leptin. So you're thin today, as a kid, a teenager, or a fortunate young adult, but you're fat tomorrow.

That's Bender's proverb.

Remember the Domino Effect of Insulin on the Hormone Cascade

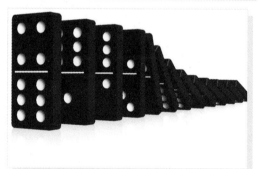

Recall that there's a domino effect to carbs. Carbs trigger insulin, which can lead to less and less sensitivity to insulin over time. When the body is no longer sensitive to insulin—"insulin resistance"—body fat builds up. The fat buildup creates other hormonal problems, as you saw in previous chapters.

The formulas are simple:

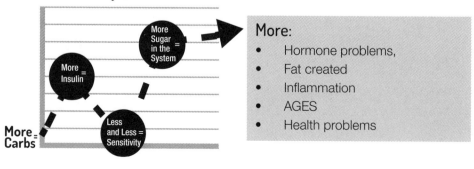

More:
- Hormone problems,
- Fat created
- Inflammation
- AGES
- Health problems

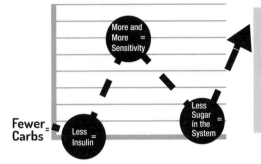

- Re-booted hormones
- Less fat
- Fewer related unhealthy signs and symptoms.

For more science on the action of insulin, go to ***Appendix III.***

The Goal of Step 2:
Go from a Sugar Burner to a Fat Burner

If you look at human history, the predominant diet was low carb. Obviously, cooked and processed grains and sugars would not have been the most dominant source of food for our forebears. We would have been eating plants (fruits in season, vegetables, some seeds and nuts) and naturally-raised and wild animals, fish, and dairy. Thus, was life in the wilderness, the frontier, or on the old farm. Carbs took off in the modern (and obese) era.

If you're going to eat like you were designed to eat—and curb the causes of obesity and aging—you can change your body's main energy source to fat.

Your brain can survive on two sources of fuel from the blood: glucose and ketones. When you eat a lot of carbohydrates, however, your brain and body become carb dependent and only utilize glucose sugar for energy. You're a sugar burner.

On the other hand, when you begin to eliminate all the sugar, you can expect your body to adapt to more fat and less sugar for energy. You become a fat burner.

Certainly you can make the argument that too much of any macronutrient calorie can kill. Yet being a fat burner comes without the metabolic shrapnel and collateral inflammatory and oxidative damage that come from excess carbs.

As you saw in previous chapters (and can see in the Appendix), you just don't find the kind of energy-related damage from burning mostly fat that you see from burning mostly sugar.

Sugar to Fat:
Making the Switch

To shift your physiology in the right direction, you generally go from higher carbs to lower carbs as your body adapts to burning fat instead of sugar. You start by finding a level of carbs in your diet that works for you and then you stay with it as your body builds back up its insulin sensitivity, reboots its hormones, and switches away from sugar and towards fat.

Just how many grams of carbs really constitute "low carb"? Here's an overview so you can see where to start.

Diets and Carbohydrate Restriction	
USDA Recommendations[42]	45–65% of total calories, or approximately 250–350 grams per day
Carbohydrate-restricted (by comparison) diet	125–200 grams per day
Moderately low-carb diet	75–100 grams per day
Very low-carbohydrate, ketogenic diet (VLCK)	40–50 grams or less per day. As little as 20g in the case of the severely insulin resistant

But let's take those numbers and make them practical—in real food terms. Here's what these amounts of carbohydrates really look like when you apply them to the real world:

Examples:

VLCK—Where Many Have to Start for Weight Loss and Re-booting Hormones.

Some stay here long term:
- 1 cup of strawberries (11g)
- 1/2 cup of almonds (15g)
- 1 avocado (12g)
- 1/2 cup of black beans (12g)

= 50g

Moderately Low

A healthy place to start or land long term depending on carb tolerance:
- 1 cup of strawberries (11g)
- sweet potato (24g)
- 1/2 cup of peanuts- (12g)
- 1/2 cup of chickpeas (27g
- 1 avocado (12g)

= 86g

Carb-Restricted

- Apple (25g)
- Cup of brown rice (45g)
- 1 cup of black beans (23g)
- 1/2 cup of almonds (15g)
- 1 cup of blueberries (21g)

= 129g

*You can visit the Carb Counter in **Chapter Eight** to find out exactly which foods can help you hit your carb target.*

As you can see, even the most carb-restricted diet could have four carbohydrate foods a day depending on portion sizes.

Most people do very well starting at the Very Low, VLCK diet. After three–four weeks, as your body adapts to burning fats, you can then move up to the Moderately Low level. Some people do so well at Very Low or are so intolerant to carbs that they stay there permanently. The "Carb-restricted diet" is really only restricted by comparison to out of control recommendations of 250–300 grams of carbs. Once you go over 125 grams per day, you have to be very active in training and high intensity sports in order to effectively utilize that much sugar.

Our doctors and patients have far and away done best starting out with the very low plan associated with our **Advanced Plan** diet. Within a few weeks, as your body adapts to burning fat, you can move to the moderately low 75–100g range and do great. Some people, however, are either so carb intolerant, or do so well on the low-carb plans, that they stay low or their weight and symptoms come back.

Young and very active people also do well with the lower end of carbohydrates in the 100–125g range available on the **Core Plan**. See our plans in **Chapter Eight**.

Tips for Determining Your Carb Tolerance

In Chapter Eight, we'll introduce you to the **Advanced** and **Core Plans**, two different carb-curbing plans that adjust to your individual level of carb tolerance.

Your carb tolerance will affect which plan is best to use to make the switch to fat burning. Here are some tips to keep in mind:

- **Diabetics and highly insulin-resistant** individuals have very little carb tolerance. In some situations, carbohydrates can even be literally toxic, which seems to suggest that a massive dietary intervention is necessary. Restricting carbohydrates to a very low-carb, ketogenic diet of around 50 grams or fewer carbohydrates per day might be necessary in order to restore insulin sensitivity and lose weight.

* *This falls under our Advanced Plan. You may need to do this just temporarily or you may find this is how you do best for the long haul.*

- **Pre-diabetics and insulin-resistant** individuals need carbohydrate restriction at 75–100 grams per day or fewer. They may need to start on the Advanced Plan. These people are not diabetic, but do have issues like high triglycerides, high blood pressure, or a high amount of abdomen fat.

* *Advanced and Core Plan*

- **Highly insulin-sensitive** people can tolerate carbohydrates for now without the need for immediate restriction, but that doesn't mean they're immune from effects in the future. Certainly a diet of 300 grams of daily carbohydrates or more is not appropriate for even the most insulin-sensitive among us.

While extremely active people, highly competitive athletes, or just the skinny freaks we hate can get away with it, it's just not a great, physiologically healthy way to live. For even the most carb tolerant, make sure you're not following a recipe for insulin resistance down the road.
* Core Plan

Chances are, you've known for a long time that you have problems that need to be dealt with—now you're getting an idea as to how extensive your carbohydrate restriction should be.

I've seen the Advanced Plan do what some believe would defy the laws of nature. Seemingly endless numbers of people are no longer diabetic after following this strategy. When my mom was sixty, she could barely walk. As a forty-eight-year smoker, she had many health problems, and the worst of them was that she couldn't go more than about twenty yards before her legs and feet hurt so much she had to sit down.

Definitions

di·a·be·tes noun \ˌdī-ə-ˈbē-tēz, -ˈbē-təs\
Type 1 Diabetes is a genetic condition in which the body cannot make insulin. In type 2 Diabetes, you may make insulin, but your cells ignore the insulin signal; i.e. you are insulin resistant – normally from several years of carb/sugar overload.

I took her to her doctor who said her issue was that she was now a diabetic. He prescribed insulin, then took us into a room where he revealed to us the horrors awaiting my mom in the future. He actually walked us through a process that would ultimately lead to amputating her legs.

That experience finally convinced my mom, who of course wouldn't listen to me. (What do I know? She changed my diapers!) But after this visit, she went full force onto the Advanced Plan and within a short period of time, the doctor removed the diagnosis of diabetes. She's seventy-two, as of this writing, and still requires no insulin and, even as New Yorker who grew up on knishes and pizza, she happily follows this way of eating and hasn't looked back.

Want More Proof Carbs Kill?

The science speaks for itself: see the Appendix on Insulin and Low-carb Diets (**Appendix III**) for research on how low-carb diets hold up when compared to low fat.

There's No Free Lunch:
The Fat-Free,
Cholesterol-Free,
Sugar-Free Debacle

My home room teacher in high school had a sign over the door that said, "There's no free lunch." Of course he meant that nothing comes easy and there are no short cuts to anyplace worth going. It takes effort—so if someone offers you a free lunch, there are strings attached.

Bread, pasta, rice, breakfast cereal, and thousands of snacks like crackers and pretzels are often labeled "fat-free, cholesterol-free, sugar-free." This is of course a marketing tactic to get the unsuspecting public buy a food product because it appears to be good for you.

The truth is, though these products really don't contain any fats, triglycerides, or cholesterol—and some don't even contain sugar—they're far from "free."

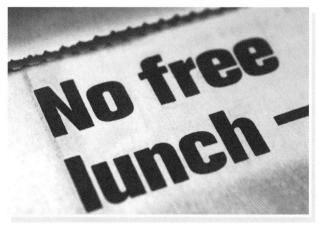

The waist-expanding problem is simple: these "fat, sugar, and cholesterol free" carbs stimulate insulin, which causes fat production. These fats then end up in a flow of triglycerides that have to be packed into cholesterol to be carried in the blood.

In other words, these "free" carbs ultimately lead to fat, triglycerides, and cholesterol.[43, 44,]

The advice to "eat carbohydrates to avoid fat" forgets that eating carbohydrates is essentially eating fat—and lots of it. The major law of Metabolics is that it's not what you eat—it's what your body makes of it.

As we've discussed, too many of these "cholesterol and triglyceride-free" carbs can create the dangerous, small LDL particles that you hear about, the "LDL pattern B," that are dangerous to your heart.

There's no free-lunch. But the great news is, when starting a low-carb diet which doesn't include these "free-foods," people will normally lower triglycerides and steadily raise HDL very quickly.[45]

A Real Test of Heart Health

The ratio of triglycerides to HDL is the most effective predictor of cardiovascular disease there is: more so than LDL/HDL ratio. Since high triglycerides are bad, and mature HDL particles are good, you want this number as low as possible: in the two or lower range. If your fasting triglycerides are greater than 150 to 500 mg/dL, you have a decreased HDL-C of less than 40 mg/dL, and an abundance of small dense LDL pattern B, which means you have a condition commonly known as "atherogenic dyslipidemia." Given what we know 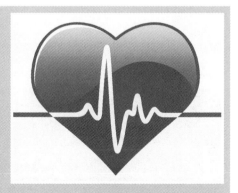 about carbohydrate and insulin action, this condition is a sign you aren't able to effectively metabolize the carbs in your diet.[46, 47]

A higher fat, low-carb diet lowers triglycerides and raises good HDL. This is an indication that you're addressing insulin resistance and heart disease which are tightly connect to this vital Triglyceride:HDL ratio.[48, 49]

More Lists of the Right Carbs to Eat
Lowering the Glycemic
Load of Your Diet

While controlling carbs, you also need to control their glycemic index. This is the degree to which your carbohydrate rich foods will drive up blood sugar. Some types of carbohydrates impact glucose levels more than others.

This becomes a greater and greater issue as your body becomes more resistant to insulin.

The glycemic index is a classification of foods, based on their impact on blood glucose levels. If the carbs are absorbed quickly, and result in a spike in insulin levels, than they have a "high glycemic index." Those foods that raise blood sugar at a slower rate, and cause less insulin release, have a lower ranking on the glycemic index.

Lower the Carbs, Raise the Sodium

Carbohydrates hold on to water and sodium in the kidneys. When you are lowering carbs, you want to add extra sodium to your diet to compensate.

The glycemic index is a measure of the increase in blood glucose when a portion of carbs, e.g., 50g of glucose or white bread, is ingested. Glucose has a GI of 100, which is a standard against which the GI of other foods is measured.

For example, if a food has a GI of 50, it can only raise blood glucose half as well as pure glucose can.

Many factors, not merely the amounts, but the type and properties of sugars, affect a food's GI. Different foods can contain a similar amount of carb grams per serving, but may impact your blood sugar in markedly different ways. It's important to know both total carbs per serving and GI.

Bottom line? Low-carb, low-GI foods are Metabolix foods.

For a complete Glycemic Index, go to the Insulin and Low-carbohydrate Diet Appendix (Appendix III).

1. Best Low-carb, Low-glycemic Index foods: These are the low-carb, low-glycemic winners.	**Examples:** Asparagus, green pepper, broccoli, Brussels sprouts, cabbage, cauliflower, celery, green beans, lettuces, mushroom, and onion are so high fiber and low GI **(10–15)** they're really "free foods"
2. Good Low-carb, Low-glycemic Index foods: Eat these foods in the morning unless you're young and/or very active.	**Examples:** Strawberries, blueberries, blackberries, raspberries **(Approx. 25)**

3. Modest-carb, Good-glycemic Index: Eat legumes in moderation. Beans are higher in carbs and GI so are best eaten mid-day with more activity left in the day to burn the carbs and more aggressive rise in sugar. Peanuts are low-carb, low Glycemic Index, but still should be eaten only once in awhile.	**Examples:** • Legumes: Peanuts.................. 7 • chickpeas............................. 10 • beans................................ **20–30**
4. Modest carb, Good Glycemic Index: Nuts and seeds	**Examples:** • Sunflower seeds................... 35 • cashews................................. 27 • almonds................................ 15 • pistachios............................. 15
5. Starchier foods, mid- to moderately high carbs and moderate Glycemic Index. Eat in moderation mid-day. Better as a lunch food, like beans, with more activity left in the day.	**Examples:** • Carrots.................................. 35 • peas....................................... 51 • sweet potato........................ 50
6. Grains, mid- to moderate carbs and high Glycemic Index. Best eaten early or when active.	**Examples:** • Brown rice............................. 50 • whole oats............................. 55
7. Grains, high carb and high Glycemic Index. For the extremely carb tolerant and active.	**Examples:** • Millet...................................... 71 • Corn.. 60 • Quinoa................................... 53
8. Off the charts. Many "healthy" foods have a higher Glycemic Index than many "junk foods" and even sugar itself. For vacation meals.	**Examples:** • Potato.........................70–100+ • White rice.............................. 89 • Instant Oatmeal..................... 83 • Oven-baked pretzels............ 83 • Cream of Wheat.................... 74 • Bagel...................................... 72 • Whole wheat bread.............. 71 • Kellogg's Special K.............. 69 **Vs. Junk Food** • White bread........................... 71 • Coca Cola.............................. 63 • Blueberry muffin.................... 60 • Ice cream, regular................. 57 • Snicker's Bar......................... 51 • Peanut M&Ms........................ 33 Note here that I'm simply making a point, not a recommendation.

GI Source: **health.harvard.edu**

Too Much Fructose

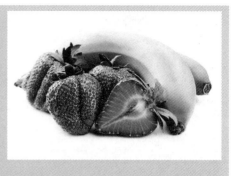

Your liver isn't designed to process the amount of fructose most people eat today. Fruit has fairly small amounts of fructose. One cup of strawberries contains 4.1 grams of fructose and 49 overall calories. You would have to eat nine cups of strawberries to get the same amount of fructose as you get in a 20 oz. soda.

A sugary fruit like a banana has 105 calories, including about 7.1 grams of fructose. Yet, you'd have to eat five bananas to get the same fructose delivery as a 20 oz. soda.

Your liver's answer to this flood of fructose is to turn most of it into fat, ship it to your fat tissue and lead to higher triglycerides and the subsequent rise of LDLs.[50]

For more on the troubles with fructose, see the ***Appendix III*** *on Insulin and Low-carbohydrates.*

But What About Fruit?

Many fruits have long enjoyed a reputation as a healthful, wholesome portion of a balanced diet. There are plenty of good reasons for this. After all, fruits come packaged with nutrients, especially vitamins. They're also a good source of dietary fiber, which has no effect on insulin and helps slow the digestion rate of the food so that the sugar isn't introduced to your system all at once.

But that doesn't mean you should load up on fruits—because the sugar will catch up to you. The best recommendation is to keep sugar to the morning, with a focus on berries, first and foremost.

Here's a quick guide to the best and worst fruits when it comes to sugar content:

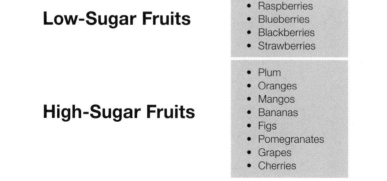

Low-Sugar Fruits

- Raspberries
- Blueberries
- Blackberries
- Strawberries

High-Sugar Fruits

- Plum
- Oranges
- Mangos
- Bananas
- Figs
- Pomegranates
- Grapes
- Cherries

Not only are berries moderate in carbs, they contain many good anti-inflammatory, anti-oxidant, anti-aging phytonutrients.

For more information on low-carb fruit, see our "Carb Counter" in ***Chapter Eight****.*

But What About Fiber?

Fiber is a carbohydrate, but since it only enters your digestive pathways (and not your metabolic pathways), it's not really even "food" and, in essence, fiber's carbs don't count.

While not a vitamin or mineral, fiber comes with benefits. For one, because it's not absorbed by your body, it won't factor in to your insulin response. This is why low carbohydrate diets don't count the carbohydrates from vegetable fiber in the daily carb tallies. These carbs are free. *For more on fiber, see **Appendix III** on Insulin and Low-carbohydrates.*

The Trouble with Wheat and Other Grains

Of all foods falling under the tenet, "carbs kill," the biggest culprits are the grains. That may be hard to imagine in a culture that celebrates, "whole grain power," the way we do. Bread packages and cereal boxes, no matter what kind of sugars, additives, or other nasty ingredients they contain, can still boast about being "Heart Healthy" if somewhere in that long list of ingredients they contain whole wheat.

Does anyone really think that Lucky Charms, Cinnamon Toast Crunch, or—for that matter—Cheerios are really health foods? Well, they're labeled that way.

Super Food, Really?

If something is whole grain, it's considered a kind of super food. But it's more likely a super killer.

You can find something good about anything. If you dig deep enough, you'll be able to come up with benefits to eating dirt, drinking from a swamp, eating leaves off of a tree, or swallowing a bug. Each likely contains some small protein or micronutrient that has value when tested in a lab or on thousands of people from out of town. But just because there's some inherent positive, doesn't mean that the ultimate outcome isn't negative.

Whole grains have fiber, certain vitamins, and minerals. For those in the inner cities of the US or in Africa who are starving, and without access to food, grains can provide life-sustaining calories.

On the other hand, there's an enormous list of colossally negative factors to grains that make them far from a health food. In the case of genetically modified grains, I'm not even sure they're a people food. While they are good fillers for those that have no food, if you're reading this book, you likely have a choice.

Grains and legumes contain elements like phytates and lectins. These are anti-nutrients. They actually block the body's ability to absorb nutrients it needs. There are beneficial lectins that you can get from following our advice to eat a moderate amount of certain grains—like brown rice and gluten-free ancient grains like amaranth. However, many lectins are extremely difficult or even impossible to assimilate and can even cause damage to digestive organs.

Soaking and sprouting help hinder some of the damaging effects of anti-nutrients, and that's how we recommend you eat your grains, legumes, and nuts. Yet, they are obviously not something to make a substantive part of your diet—and standard commercial products don't use sprouted grains, so the issues are still intact.

See how to soak and sprout in **Appendix IX**.

The Problem with Wheat	The main grain people eat is wheat. Or at least what we still call wheat. The current product is a distant gene-spliced, child-of-two-first-cousins kind of food. The increased consumption of this product has run completely parallel to the population getting sicker and fatter. Grains all have similar problems; wheat is just the most common and arguably the worst. In addition to the anti-nutrients, there's also the way the human condition reacts to the current evolution of grain products.
Gluten	Gluten-free products, ranging from cookies to crackers, have become extremely popular. Gluten is a protein found in grains like wheat, barley, and rye and is added to many, many foods. Some combination of the genetic modification of grains, carb levels, and gluten has been proven to cause a terrible reaction in many people. Celiac disease, diabetes, heart disease, arthritis, and even mental and emotional issues are now just some of the serious and even life-threatening auto-immune diseases tied to eating gluten and other dangerous components of wheat and other gluten grains. The gluten-free product, however, leaves a lot to be desired. Most of them are highly refined foods where the wheat is replaced with high carb, high glycemic grains and starches, like white rice, potato, and corn. You end up trading one devil for another. There are many great books and programs out there that dive deeper into the issue of wheat, gluten, and genetically modified organisms (GMOs). A quick web search, and you'll be inundated with this information.
Genetically Modified Organisms (GMOs)	What are GMOS? These foods have had their DNA changed. It's "refined food on steroids." There's great concern about both the current and future well-being of the public and how people will respond to eating food mutations. **Common GMOs include:** Soy, canola, sugar beets, corn, wheat, tomatoes, and potatoes. There are additional concerns that the eggs, dairy products, and meats derived from animals eating GMOs may be negatively impacted. These make me think of movies like Terminator or Legend where the world has ended due to some apocalyptically bad scientific decision. As Schwarzenegger would say, "Stay away from GMOs if you want to live."

What Grains Can I Eat?

There are reports that "ancient grains" are available that are not genetically modified and are gluten-free. While these would still be high in carbs and on the glycemic index, you'd avoid these other dangers. As grains, they don't qualify as food, but are allowed in moderation on our Core Plan.

Gluten-free ancient grains: Amaranth, quinoa, buckwheat, and millet

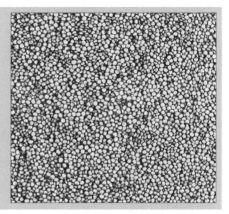

Legumes and Nuts

Beans and legumes may be tolerated reasonably well by some people; however, they cause problems for many others. They are similar to grains in their ability to develop toxins against mammals, and they must be cooked or sprouted before eating.

Beans contain the lectin phytohaemagglutin and alpha-amylase inhibitor, which block the digestion of stomach acid and prevent the proper digestion and assimilation of nutrients.[51, 52, 53] Beans are notoriously difficult to digest and absorb due to their high galacto-oligosaccharides content, which often results in abdominal pain, bloating, and gas. While beans are high in fiber, they are also fairly high in non-fiber carbohydrate.

Although nuts also have lectins, they appear to be fewer in number and less harmful than those found in grains and beans; for instance, nuts can be consumed raw with no deleterious effects, while eating uncooked grains or beans could result in serious illness. Nuts are also low in non-fiber carbohydrates and provide healthy fats. When consumed in small amounts, nuts should pose little harm to health.

To make these foods better and safer to consume, again, be sure to follow the soaking instructions found in **Appendix IX**.

Sweet Sensations and Sugar Substitutes:
Can You Have Your Cake
and Eat It, Too?

Breaking up with sweets is hard to do. For me, my family, and most of our patients around the world, we find we're married to the taste of sweetness for life. The key is to learn how to manage carbs without going so overboard that the excess energy kills you—and without poisoning yourself with toxic sweeteners.

One common fear people have about the low carb diet is that they'll never get to taste anything sweet again. But remain calm! I eat two to three "desserts" every day. These desserts are delicious and leave you without the cravings for sugar. The secret? Make your desserts without grain flours, sugars, or artificial sweeteners.

It is possible to have tasty, sweet desserts on the low-carb diet—even baked goods. Just pay attention to The Natural, The Good, The Not-As-Good, and The Ugly.

The Natural	Natural sweeteners such as **raw, organic honey, maple syrup**, and **coconut sugar** allow you the flavor you're looking for, without the toxic effects. Additionally, while sugar is literally an anti-nutrient, these have some nutritional value. On the other hand, as you count the carbs and begin to measure whether or not you're in excess, realize that natural sweeteners have much of the same ultimate metabolic effect as sugar itself. So these are to be limited and better used in the case of the very active lifestyle and intense workout recovery.
The Good	**Stevia**, a South American herb, doesn't appear to cause any harmful effects based on existing studies; in fact, it may potentially improve blood pressure and blood glucose control, although findings have not been universal in this regard.[54] Stevia can be used to sweeten anything—plain yogurt, smoothies, and is heat stable so it works in coffee, tea, and baked goods. Certain brands taste better than others. Pure stevia products and liquid extracts are preferable to granular formulations like Truvia and Purevia, which contain dextrose (sugar).
The Not-As-Good	**Xylitol** tends to have less of a laxative effect than the other types and in addition may be beneficial for dental health in large quantities—and large quantities are not recommended. The source of xylitol and the processing required to make it doesn't make this a natural or whole food. It is good for baking, so use sparingly where dessert recipes warrant. **The sugar alcohols**. While there is no evidence of harmful effects from sugar alcohols, they can cause gastrointestinal upset such as gas, bloating, or diarrhea.[55] **Erythritol** is the only sugar alcohol that has a negligible effect on blood sugar levels, and extensive research demonstrates that it is safe for human consumption.[56] Erythritol is equal in sweetness to sugar, with a very similar texture and taste, making it ideal for baked goods. **Malitol, mannitol, and sorbitol.** These sugar alcohols are partially absorbed by the small intestine and do contribute calories (about half as much as sucrose) and can impact blood sugar in people with diabetes, unless consumed in very small quantities.

The Ugly

Sugar Substitutes: Although the FDA's position is that the sweeteners below are safe if consumed in moderate amounts, there is disturbing research about these chemicals.

Sucralose research has resulted in contradictory findings. Although early research indicated that sucralose was safe, one study found altered gut flora in animals consuming the sweetener.[57]

Aspartame has had many reports of adverse effects in users, primarily headaches, difficulty concentrating, and memory loss. There are several independent studies implicating aspartame in fibromyalgia[61], memory loss[62], cancer[63], and weight gain.[58, 59, 60, 61]

Saccharin is an intense sweetener, which is about five hundred times sweeter than sucrose, and can be toxic in high doses.[62]

Maltodextrin is a food additive derived from starches, and it's an ingredient present in processed foods all across your grocery store. Because it is processed in your body as glucose, it's not a good way to sweeten your foods. It's also highly processed, usually coming from carbs like corn and potato.

"Yogi Berra Math"

"Baseball is ninety percent mental. The other half is physical."

-Yogi Berra

Just do the math. The calories have to come from somewhere. So if the recommendation is low fat and low protein, then all that's left is carbs.

The maximum, modern recommendation for fat in your diet is 30% fat, and government

Chocolate Avocado Pudding *(one serving)*

Ingredients
- 1 avocado, soft and ripe
- 1 teaspoon vanilla
- 1/4 cup cocoa powder
- stevia to taste
- 6 tablespoons coconut milk
- 1/4 cup of ice *(Even better with a scoop of Perfect Protein)*

Directions
1. Cut avocado in half and remove pit. Scoop out flesh and put it in the blender along with remaining ingredients.
2. Process until smooth, occasionally scraping down sides. Serve immediately or refrigerate until ready to serve. *Ice keeps it from getting hot in the blender so you can eat it right away.*

allowances for protein are only around 15–20%. So even as the rope is being let out slightly on fat recommendations, over 50% of the diet still remains carbs! Only the most carb tolerant can stay lean or even survive these recommendations.

The bottom line is that the low-fat, high carb diet era has gone hand in hand with skyrocketing rates of obesity and diabetes and the continual epidemic of cardiovascular disease. Get used to over 50% of your calories coming from fat.

Key Concepts From This Chapter

1. Controlling insulin starts with controlling carbs.

Yes, protein can have an insulin effect, but carbohydrates (particularly high-GI carbohydrates) have the greatest effect on blood sugar and insulin. If you want to stay lean and prevent the metabolic damage wreaked by chronically high insulin, you'll have to start controlling the carbs in your diet.

2. Fructose is an especially dangerous sweetener.

It's not so prevalent in fiber and nutrient-rich fruits, but it's prevalent in the soft drinks you'll find at the grocery store. Even many breads come packed with high-fructose corn syrup these days. If you want to stay healthy, avoid fructose in high amounts.

3. You can still eat sweet things.

In the Maximized Metabolix diet, you'll be able to eat desserts! But you have to use the right sweeteners. In the final appendix of this book, you'll get the recipes for creating baked goods and sweets that don't have the sugar load of most desserts, thereby allowing you to diet without all the sacrifice.

4. "Bender's Proverb."

Just because you aren't fat today doesn't mean that excess carbohydrates in your diet won't wreak havoc in your long-term future. If you want to prevent aging and inflammation, you have to keep insulin under control. The most powerful tool for this is keeping your carbs under control. Don't be "skinny today, but fat tomorrow."

CHAPTER FIVE:

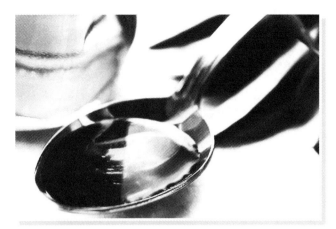

Oil Change:
Change the Priority of Fats in Your Diet

H2A2 Formula Step 2

Must-have fats in your kitchen:

- Dark, unsweetened chocolate bars
- Unsweetened cocoa powder
- Fish—-wild-caught sardines, herring, and salmon
- Fish oil capsules or liquid
- Chia seeds
- Flax seeds
- Avocado
- Almonds
- Pecans
- Pistachios
- Organic Almond butter

- Organic peanut butter
- Extra virgin olive oil
- Extra virgin coconut oil
- Organic, grass-fed butter *(Raw is best—at least do organic, as toxins stick to fats)*
- Coconut flour
- Almond flour
- Coconut milk
- Whole olives
- Coconut oil
- Organic, grass, and finished fed meats

Don't be Scared

When my youngest son turned four, he learned how to manipulate people (or at least attempt to) by challenging their will. If someone said they didn't want to play a particular game, or his sister wouldn't share her drink, he'd say, "Why, are you scared?"

Once, when my family was taking a cab home from the airport, the driver was listening to the news. My son, apparently not liking this choice of entertainment, asked if the cab driver could change the station. When the driver said he couldn't because the company doesn't let him, my son responded, "Come on, don't be scared."

When you restrict your carbs, you'll be getting more calories from fat. But don't be scared! As we established in previous chapters, it's not dietary fat that makes your butt look fat, clogs your arteries, and packs onto your hips and thighs.

Fats Out of Order

Fat is good, but we have to change the amounts of which fats you eat.

Modern society has you getting the mass majority of your fats from omega-6s, eating too many trans-fats, and getting very, very little from omega-3s.

It's also likely that you're eating a lot of commercially raised animal products which contain toxins and a poor, unbalanced assortment of fats.

Monounsaturated fats from whole foods like extra virgin olive oil and raw almonds are lacking in many diets. For some, there's an overemphasis on monos, which can be found in body fat, and an under-emphasis on MCTs from coconut oil that aren't.

When it all comes down to it, you may be in need of an "oil change."

What's Wrong with Most Peoples' Current Fats

Omega-6s	Way Too Many
Omega-3s	Far Too Few
Commercial Animal Fats	Too Many
Naturally Pasture-Raised and Fed Animal Fats and CLA	Nearly Non-Existent
Monounsaturated Fats	Too Few
MCTs	Too Few
Synthetic Trans Fats	Any is Too Many

The Oil Change

- Radically reduce omega-6 fats.
- Increase omega-3 fats from flax and chia seeds and highly unsaturated DHA and EPA from the list of safe fish and fish oils, you'll find in the chapter "iProtein."
- Add monounsaturated fats found in olive oil, avocado, raw nuts and seeds.
- Use MCTs from coconut oil, coconut flour and coconut milk.
- Eat clean saturated fats from pasture-raised cows and chickens along with dairy products and eggs.
- The pasture raised cows supply more CLA (conjugated linoleic acid).
- Avoid trans-fats.

What will your kitchen look like when you've made the changes, above?

- Reduce the 6s: roasted nuts, vegetable, nut, or seed oils in packaged and prepared foods, reduce/eliminate commercial meat and dairy products.
- Add the 3s: Chia or flax seeds in yogurt, smoothies, or on salads; wild-caught salmon or sardines, others from the safe fish list; green vegetables; and an omega supplement
- •Add monounsaturated (omega-9) fats: Extra virgin olive oil on salads instead of commercial dressings; avocados, a couple of handfuls of almonds, almond flour, hazelnuts, or macadamia nuts.
- Medium chain triglycerides: Coconut milk in your smoothies, cook at moderate heat with coconut oil, recipes using coconut flour.
- Add saturated fats from good, clean sources. Although higher in monounsaturated fats than saturated—grass-fed, grass finished hamburger or steak, pasture raised and organic chicken and eggs, organic, grass-fed cheese and butter (raw is best if possible). Adds CLA as well.

There you have it: a simple formula for changing your life. Now, let me explain why it works.

Fat:
The Misunderstood
Macronutrient

Fat burns cleaner than other fuels. In fact, certain fats help you to actually burn body fat, and they support many of your body's most critical functions.

Another old food misnomer is the idea of eating "good fat." This is really a concept designed for the outmoded *fat = cholesterol = heart disease* theory where "good fats" were those that lowered LDL cholesterol.

With both time and maturing science, this theory has dramatically changed.

Flip Your Old Thinking Upside Down

Rather than view fat as "bad," realize it is actually your body's preferred fuel source. Given that fact, the concept of *"low fat = healthy"* may be the poorest nutritional recommendation in history.

Consider that many of the fats you eat go on to make up your body's cells and tissues. Perhaps most importantly, they make up the outer layer of your cells (the membrane). This outer membrane, which orchestrates much of inner cellular health, requires a particular balance of the different fats that make it up.

Body tissues are made up of many fatty acids. These include **saturated palmitic acid, monounsaturated oleic acid, and the omega-3, 6, and 9 highly unsaturated fatty acids (HUFAs)**. So most fats are critical to your cells and body function. As strange as it sounds, to be truly healthy, you need to eat a variety of different kinds of fats. What's important is that you get your fats in the right balance.

The Critical Omega-3 and Omega-6 Fat Balance

There are two types of fatty acids that your body can't synthesize on its own: omega-3s and omega-6s. This makes them essential nutrients, which means you can't live without consuming both.

Too much omega-6 will drive down the presence and influence of important omega-3s and omega-9s. In fact, the omega-9 HUFA is thought by some to be a metabolic toxin when it is really a biomarker (measurement) of potentially beneficial restricted intake of omega-6.

This balance is critically important because these two fats take different paths in your body:

Omega-3s	Omega-6s
The omega-3 PUFAs become the highly unsaturated fatty acids (HUFAs) known as EPA and DHA. This path is anti-inflammatory.	The omega-6s become highly unsaturated arachidonic acid (AA). This path is inflammatory.

Why is this important? The amount of HUFA in the body is finite. This creates a big metabolic challenge as the 3s and 6s compete with each other for the enzymes and "shelf space" in your membranes. Therefore, too many omega-6s will overtake the omega-3s in your tissues and leave you in the unhealthy and unhappy inflammatory state.

These large amounts of omega-6 fatty acids largely come from vegetable, corn, soybean, and nut oils—along with commercial animal products. For example, corn oil contains forty-six times more omega-6 than 3.[64]

The famous MRFIT study and studies of many different cultures show that people with the lowest percentage of omega-6s in HUFA had the lowest death rate.[65] In fact, as other cultures like Japan become more westernized and their percentage of omega-6s goes up, we can observe rapidly growing levels of cardiovascular disease.[66, 67, 68]

Keeping the Balance

It is vital not to let your omega-6 levels dwarf omega 3s. Yet this is exactly what has occurred. The average American eats between ten and thirty times more omega-6 fatty acids than omega-3 fatty acids, leaving their systems with 80% omega-6 compared to 20% omega-3.[63] Many healthier cultures have a 60% omega-6 to 40% omega-3 balance.

Remember: omega-6s are essential to your body. You just don't need that much of them. You only need somewhere between a half of a percent[69] of your entire calorie intake to three percent of your entire fat calorie intake to meet your daily need.

Omega Balance, Disease, and Inflammation

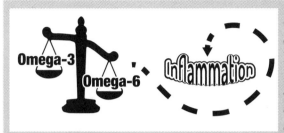

Omega-6 fats lead to the formation of "eicosanoids." This is a group of hormones involved in your body's inflammatory process. When omega-6 levels get high, the body can go into a state of chronic and dangerous inflammation, leading to cardiovascular disease and other severe conditions and diseases. In fact, the action that allows many painkillers, like aspirin, to work is the inhibition of the enzymes that convert omega-6 to inflammatory agents (called prostaglandins).[70]

Over time, it's been estimated that the overabundance of omega-6s and the resulting deficiency of omega-3s is involved in the causes of heart disease, vascular disease, homicide, depression, bronchial disease, and many other brain, joint, and organ disorders.[71, 72, 73, 74]

The omega-3s in your body can compete for, slow down, and even stop the formation of these inflammatory omega-6 hormones. This fact led to the discovery that increasing omega-3 HUFAs as a percent of your body's lipids could prevent diseases caused by omega-6 inflammation.[75, 76]

In all, the science has shown a number of benefits to health and wellness when you get enough omega-3 fatty acids in your diet:

Getting Enough Omega-3s: Potential Health Benefits	
Weight loss	Omega-3 fatty acids can be beneficial in weight loss.[77]
Lowering Triglycerides	The Mayo Clinic says there is "strong scientific evidence from human trials" that omega-3 fatty acids from fish help lower triglyceride levels, which lowers cardiovascular disease risk
Rheumatoid Arthritis	Omega-3 fatty acids can be beneficial for joints, helping prevent rheumatoid arthritis.[78] Hypertension, Although the reductions are modest, the evidence for a link between better blood pressure and omega-3 fatty acids is strong.[79]

Stroke	Some evidence suggests that omega-3s are protective against stroke as well as arterial-wall buildup.[80]
Acute Coronary Syndrome	This type of heart disease has been associated with low levels of omega-3 fatty acids.[81]
Cancer	Omega-3 fatty acids were shown to attenuate growth and induce apoptosis in a variety of human cancer cell lines derived from colonic, pancreatic, prostate, and breast cancer.[82]
Psychiatric Benefits	Depression, post-partum depression, homicide, bi-polar disorder, and many behavioral problems have been linked to low omega-3s.[83]

Omega-3 and Omega-6
Polyunsaturated Fatty Acids in Your Diet

Now that you know what these fatty acids do in your body, let's take a second to examine exactly what they are—and where you can find them.

First, let's list the omega-3 fatty acids commonly found in the diet:

Better Weight Loss and Body Composition With Omega-3s

There's a mechanism through which increasing the intake of omega 3 PUFA could improve body composition. It does this by causing increased fat breakdown in cardiac, adipose, liver, intestinal, and muscle tissue, leading to reduced fat storage in the body. Additionally, studies show that omega-3s can increase lean tissue mass, therefore potentially increasing metabolism and reducing body fat this way, as well.

What's more, there is evidence from studies that adequate omega 3 fatty acid intake might also further reduce the feelings of hunger after eating.[344]

ALA: Alpha-linolenic acid	Found in flax and chia seeds and in vegetables. Also occurs in hemp seeds and walnuts, but as you'll see, hemp seeds and walnuts contain a high quantity of linoleic acid so are really better defined as sources of omega-6 linoleic vs. omega-3 ALA.
EPA: Eicosapentaenoic acid	Typically found in marine food sources like fatty fish.
DHA: Docosahexaenoic acid	Typically found in marine food sources like fatty fish.

Humans can convert ALAs into EPA and DHAs, but we're not very good at it when we eat lots of competing omega-6 fats. That's why you need to make it a point to get all of these omega-3s in your diet.

As for omega-6 essential fatty acids, let's take a close look at linoleic acid. It's an essential nutrient, but overly available so deficiency isn't a concern. Over-consumption is.

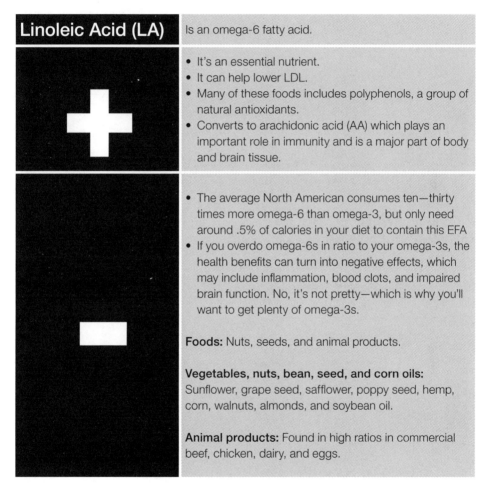

Linoleic Acid (LA)	Is an omega-6 fatty acid.

- It's an essential nutrient.
- It can help lower LDL.
- Many of these foods includes polyphenols, a group of natural antioxidants.
- Converts to arachidonic acid (AA) which plays an important role in immunity and is a major part of body and brain tissue.

- The average North American consumes ten—thirty times more omega-6 than omega-3, but only need around .5% of calories in your diet to contain this EFA
- If you overdo omega-6s in ratio to your omega-3s, the health benefits can turn into negative effects, which may include inflammation, blood clots, and impaired brain function. No, it's not pretty—which is why you'll want to get plenty of omega-3s.

Foods: Nuts, seeds, and animal products.

Vegetables, nuts, bean, seed, and corn oils: Sunflower, grape seed, safflower, poppy seed, hemp, corn, walnuts, almonds, and soybean oil.

Animal products: Found in high ratios in commercial beef, chicken, dairy, and eggs.

What's Your Score? Omega-3 and Omega-6 Balance Scores

How do you achieve an adequate balance of omega-3s and omega-6s in your body? The balance of these fats in your body correlates with the balance in your diet.

The oil in fish contains large amounts of EPA and DHA, and arachidonic acid can be found directly in animal products. To cut back on the 6 and increase the 3, one of the most important nutritional numbers to track is your omega-3 to omega-6 balance score.

Not that I want to give you yet another variable to track and measure all day. But this balance is an extremely important dynamic. You'll want your score to be as positive as possible in your fight to slow down aging and prevent disease.

For this score, you're looking for foods with a positive or plus (+) in front of them and not a minus (-). While some foods contain omega-3s, if they also contain a whole lot of omega-6s, then they still have a negative (-) omega-3 balance score.

The more negative the score, the more inflammatory omega-6 you have. +3 is anti-inflammatory.

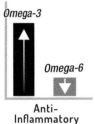

Omega-Positive Fats (+ Omega-3)

Flax seeds and **chia seeds** have high levels of omega-3 PUFAs and are (+32) and (+24) respectively. Add fresh crushed flax seeds and whole chia seeds to everything.

Fish is the richest source of omega-3 fatty acids and contains the HUFAs EPA and DHA, which means they don't have to be converted inside your body. Mackerel, for example, is a +109 and salmon a +73.

The goal is to eat fish two–three days a week. However, the challenge of finding clean sources of wild (and not toxic, farm-raised) fish makes this difficult. See the list of best and worst fish to eat in "iProtein."

"Good" Fats with Negative (- omega-3) Scores.

Some foods containing what are called "good fats" may surprise you with their negative scores.

Olive oil and **avocado** are each -10. A -10 isn't that bad and is easily made up for by adding +3 foods.

Bacon and lard—although they are not foods on our recommended list, it may shock you to know that they actually have similar fatty acid profiles to olive oil and avocados, are a -10.

If you're old enough, you remember when the music artist Prince changed his name to a symbol. As a result, when he was announced, they'd say, "The artist formerly known as Prince."

What we'll call the fats "formally known as good fats" are the nuts and seeds. They were known as good fats because they were high in omega-6 PUFAs.

Fats Formally Known as Good Fats

Cashews are -14 and almonds are -21.

Pumpkin seeds are -38, **sunflower seeds** are -39, and **safflower** are -54. Yikes!

What's more, if you roast your sunflower seeds in omega-6 vegetable oil they rate a -58. Roasting also heats the PUFAs, which causes them to oxidize. More on fat oxidation in this chapter.

The most shocking negative scores come from foods known as quality sources of omega-3s. The problem? Too high a ratio of omega-6s:

Walnuts: black (-50) and English (-44)

Hemp oil: (-39)

Grape-seed oil is also "touted" healthy, but its score (-79) suggests otherwise

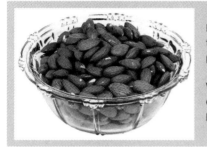

Oh, Nuts!

Nuts and seeds are high in omega-6s. On the other hand, they are mostly low-carb, low glycemic, whole foods that provide natural proteins and other quality nutrients.

While they shouldn't make up a high percent of your daily diet, a couple of handfuls a day can help you find a good, low-carb snack and provide other good health benefits.

Vegetables

Many vegetables are great sources of omega 3s.

Seaweed provides up to a +25 score in addition to being the only plant that contains DHA and EPA directly.

Spinach, lettuces, broccoli, cauliflower, squash, and Brussels sprouts are all decent sources of ALA, ranging from +1 to +4.

Meat and Dairy

Beef is a -1 to a -2 and chicken a -2 to -4.

Milk is a 0 and eggs are upwards of a -17.

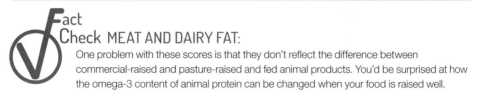

Fact Check MEAT AND DAIRY FAT:

One problem with these scores is that they don't reflect the difference between commercial-raised and pasture-raised and fed animal products. You'd be surprised at how the omega-3 content of animal protein can be changed when your food is raised well.

Grain-fed, commercial cows accumulate more omega-6 in their tissues than naturally grass-fed cows and have much lower omega-3s.[84]

Similarly, chickens raised in the pasture, getting sunlight and eating their natural diet of greens and bugs, contain higher levels of omega-3s in their meat and eggs than the un-natural, feed-fed chickens raised on corn and soy.[85]

To view the 6-3 balance score of hundreds of foods in your diet, go to http://www.fastlearner. org/omega3-6balance.htm

How Many Omega-3s Should You Get?

If you want to know more about how many omega-3s you should get as a baseline, refer to the chart below:

Life stage	Expert Recommendations for the Adequate Intake (AI) of Omega-3s
Pregnancy	**DHA:** • minimum of 300 mg / day
Lactation	**DHA:** • minimum of 300 mg / day
Infancy	**DHA (mother's intake):** • 200–300 mg / day
Childhood	**EPA + DHA combined:** • 1–3 years old: 70 mg • 4–8 years old: 90 mg • 9–13 years old: 120 mg **ALA:** • 1–3 years old: 700 mg • 4–8 years old: 900 mg • 9–13 years old: 1,200 mg
Adulthood	**EPA + DHA combined:** • 650 mg / day • Minimum 220 mg / day from EPA • Minimum 220 mg / day from DHA
Aging	**EPA + DHA combined:** • 650 mg - 700 mg / day • Minimum 220 mg / day from EPA • Minimum 220 mg / day from DHA **ALA:** • Elderly men: 1,600 mg • Elderly women: 1,100 mg

As it's unlikely you'll get the amount of omega-3s needed from your diet alone, supplementation is usually necessary.

Should You Seek Out Omega-3 Supplements?

Health Status	AHA Recommendations
Adults with coronary heart disease	Take fish oil omega-3 supplements under doctor supervision; 1 gram daily of EPA and DHA.
Adults with high cholesterol	Take fish oil omega-3 supplements under doctor supervision; 2–4 grams daily of EPA and DHA
Adults with high blood pressure	Take omega-3 supplements under doctor supervision; 3–4 grams daily of EPA and DHA

One final caveat about omega-3s and omega-6s: it's generally hard do without supplementation, but people who are too diligent about their omega balance can drive the 6s too low and the 3s too high. Omega-6s are important for brain growth and development in the fetus, newborn, and beyond.

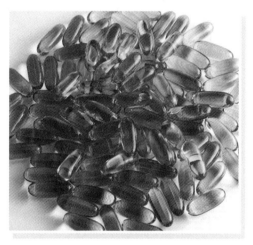

As with omega-6, people are rarely deficient in GLA (omega-6 gamma linoleic acid) or omega-9 fats, as you acquire or make these on your own from commonly eaten foods.

The best—and a highly recommended—way to learn your omega balances is to consult with your doctor and have your blood tested through a simple finger-prick profile.

Know Your Fats and Oils

Now that you know where to find omega-3s, both in your diet and in supplements, it's time to talk about the rest of the fats you get in your diet.

Mono-unsaturated Fats

Monounsaturated fats are found in oils, nuts, and avocados, as many people know. What may surprise you is that they're also found in high quantities in animal sources like whole butter, beef, eggs, and chicken.

Oleic Acid

Oleic acid, an omega-9, is renowned for its favorable effects on blood cholesterol markers.

Olive oil and avocados, in particular, are rich, healthy sources of oleic acid that have been shown to promote a number of positive health effects.

Good food sources:
- Beef, butter, poultry, eggs, human breast milk, avocados, almonds, macadamias, and hazelnuts (filberts)
- Vegetable oils: Olive, macadamia nut oil, high-oleic sunflower oil

Health Comments

Inhibits inflammation, which helps explain a reduced risk of cardiovascular disease (CVD)

Often comes from food sources rich in polyphenols, a group of natural antioxidants that may help increase longevity

Helps improve health markers related to diabetes, including those related to CVD risk

Oleic acid is the primary monounsaturated fat in the standard human diet. However, palmintoleic acid, an omega-7, can be found in sources like macadamia oil, and has shown similar benefits to insulin sensitivity.

Here are some tips on getting the health benefits of monounsaturated fats while balancing out your omega profile:

1 Don't Overdo It

People will often overdo monounsaturated fats since they've been called the "good fat" for so many years.

Like with many fats, there are real benefits. But also, these are fats found in the fat you don't want in your body, stored in your belly and thighs.

2 Improve Your Omega Score

IMPORTANT!

While many monos have positive benefits, they have more 6 than 3 and a score of -10. By adding flax or chia seeds to meals containing foods like avocado and olive oil, you can up omega-3 levels.

Many food sources of monounsaturated fat have benefits beyond their overall healthy fat. Olive oil, avocados, and almonds contain phytochemicals that can reduce inflammation and help you fight disease.

Polyunsaturated Fats

Gamma-linolenate:
A Conditionally Essential Fatty Acid

Gamma-linolenate (GLA) is an important PUFA, an omega-6 and a product of linolenic acid. It's also a conditionally essential fatty acid because of our hampered ability to convert linolenic acid to dihomo-γ-linolenic acid (DGLA). This challenge has been correlated with everything from hormonal issues in women to aging and cancer.

Found in borage and evening primrose oil, this fat has been found to help obese patients keep the weight off.[86] This is why some people are required to supplement with GLA, as well, and get great benefits from products containing sources like evening primrose and borage.

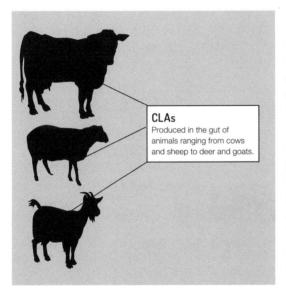

CLAs
Produced in the gut of animals ranging from cows and sheep to deer and goats.

The Health Benefits of Conjugated Linoleic Acids (CLAs)
Conjugated linoleic acids, or CLAs, are garnering some well-earned attention for their potential health benefits.

Conjugated linoleic acids are a group of isomers to linoleic acid, an essential nutrient. They're produced in the gut of animals ranging from cows and sheep to deer and goats. You can also find CLAs in the dairy and meat products that come from these animals.

What's so great about CLAs? The science is beginning to show a number of benefits, including:

Anti-cancer properties. CLAs are anti-carcinogenic, leading some studies to hypothesize direct CLA treatment may even help fight cancer. Many animal studies have revealed that treatment with CLAs can even help reduce the size of tumors.[87]

Benefits in weight management. An analysis of CLA studies in humans[88] concluded that doses of CLAs overall produced a "modest loss in body fat mass" independent of other variables. In the study, 3.2 grams per day produced ninety grams of fat lost in one week, which is statistically significant.

This is another great reason to go "wild" when it comes to your meats. CLA is found in much greater quantities in naturally, grass-fed animals. More on the raising of animals in "iProtein."

Saturated Fats

There are three categories of saturated fats: short-chain, medium-chain, and long-chain fatty acids. Let's look at them in greater detail:

Short-Chain Fatty Acids (SCFAs

The primary short-chain fatty acid in the human diet is butyric acid, which is Greek for butter.

Because short-chain fatty acids are easily absorbed into your body, they are not normally turned to body fat.

Foods: Butter, coconut oil, palm kernel oil, Parmesan cheese, milk (especially goat and sheep milk)

Health Comments

- Burned quickly for energy
- Lower in calories than long-chain fatty acids
- Colon health and protection[89]
- Links to anti-inflammatory effects
- Have been used to treat Crohn's disease[90]
- Improved cell health in the small and large intestines

Health Comments

- Burned quickly for energy
- Lower in calories than long-chain fatty acids
- Anti-microbial
- Potential anti-aging properties
- Used frequently by athletes as supplements for burning fat and retaining lean mass
- Can help with appetite control, making them highly useful for fat loss.
- They've even been used for treatment in cycstic fibrosis, Alzheimer's disease, and childhood seizures.[91]
- Inhibits inflammation, which helps explain a reduced risk of cardiovascular disease (CVD)
- Includes polyphenols, a group of natural antioxidants
- Helps improve health markers for sufferers of diabetes, including CVD risk

Medium-Chain Fatty Acids (MCFAs)

Lauric acid, a medium-chain triglyceride found in human breast milk and coconut products.

Foods: Coconut oil, palm kernel oil

NOTE: Due to its mode of digestion, it's the best fat to use for those without a gallbladder or with gallbladder issues.

Health Comments

Long-Chain Fatty Acids (LCFAs)

Many long-chain fatty acids can be found in the typical human diet. For example, stearic acid is the most common fat found in plants and animals. Palmitic acid is even more common when you include all of nature.

Foods: Palm oil, shortening, lard, tallow, butter, pork and beef fat, cottonseed oil

- Stearic acid, in particular, is associated with lowering LDL cholesterol[92]
- Palmitic acid is a major lung surface substance, aiding in lung protection and the immune system
- Your body can make palmitic and stearic acid from carbohydrates in the diet. This is critical, as reducing fat intake does not necessarily mean you're not adding on saturated fat!

Common Saturated Fatty Acids in the Diet

Saturated fats like lauric acid and stearic acid don't go rancid or become oxidized easily. This is good and makes them more stable to store and use for cooking.

Other saturated fats to be aware of include:

Lauric acid	Is the anti-microbial, anti-fungal, anti-bacterial fat in Coconut oil and human breast milk that helps keep babies healthy.
Myristic acid	a saturated fat found in butter and coconut oil, was shown to have positive effects on cholesterol in a 2005 study[93]. This effect was mostly found to be associated with a moderate intake of the fat.
Stearic acid	Stearic Acid, a fat with uses beyond nutrition like the making of soaps, shampoos, and shaving creams, is another fat produced by the metabolism of carbohydrates. It enjoys a reputation amongst the satured fats as having high potential cholesterol-friendly effects.[94]

But Doesn't Saturated Fat Give You Heart Disease?

Thus far, you've been reading a lot about increasing healthy fats—and, yes, I've included saturated fats in this group. If you've experienced a few internal warning sirens every time saturated fatty acids have been mentioned as "good" sources of fat, you're not alone. One of the most pervasive food myths is that eating more saturated fat will give you heart disease.

Much of the "saturated fat =heart disease" myth rose out of the early belief that total cholesterol was a strong indicator of heart disease risk. Because saturated fat can raise total cholesterol, HDL along with LDL, much of the recent science has taken a more nuanced approach to SFAs.

Let's put the fear of all saturated fats to rest:

A Scientific Look at Saturated Fat and Heart Disease

Study	Year	Comments
Dietary fiber and saturated fat intake associations with cardiovascular disease differ by sex in the Malmö Diet and Cancer Cohort: a prospective study.[95]	2012	A low-carbohydrate, high-fat diet produced "favorable effects on body weight and major cardiovascular risk factors."
Meta-analysis of prospective cohort studies evaluating the association of saturated fat with cardiovascular disease	2010	Meta-study reviewing over 300,000 subjects finds "saturated fat is not associated with an increased risk of CHD or CVD."
A systematic review of the evidence supporting a causal link between dietary factors and coronary heart disease.	2009	"Insufficient evidence" that saturated and polyunsaturated fatty acid intake are correlated with heart disease.
Long term effects of ketogenic diet in obese subjects with high cholesterol level.[96]	2006	An examination of a low-carbohydrate, high-fat diet finds that HDL increased while triglycerides, LDL, and total cholesterol decreased.
The questionable role of saturated and polyunsaturated fatty acids in cardiovascular disease.	1998	Saturated and polyunsaturated fats not correlated with increased risks of heart disease; in one cohort, total fat is inversely correlated with heart disease.
Effect of dietary fatty acids on serum lipids and lipoproteins.	1992	Meta analysis of 27 separate diet trials finds that saturated fats raise HDL.

If you're still unsure about eating saturated fat, consider the Framingham Heart Study, an ongoing cardiovascular study of the town of Framingham, Massachusetts.

Examining thousands of subjects over a period of decades, the former study director, Dr. William P. Castelli, wrote in the Journal of the American Medical Association: "The more saturated fat one ate, the more cholesterol one ate, the more calories one ate, the lower the person's serum cholesterol."[97]

While it will take time for the mainstream headlines to start catching up with the science of saturated fat, don't believe all the hype.

On the other hand, while changing out saturated fats for carbs has clearly been a terrible idea, loading up on saturated fats isn't the ideal. Rather than carbs as a saturated fat replacement, going to vegetables, omega-3 foods, lower-carb and glycemic foods, and a moderate amount of legumes is the way to go.

Food Sources of Fats

Knowing which fats to eat is not enough—you have to know where to get them. Let's look at some of the most common fat sources in the human diet and identify specifically which fats comprise their dietary fat.

Food	Saturated Fat	Unsaturated Fat	Chief Fat Sources
Dairy			
Butter	61%	33%	31% Palmitic, 24% Oleic 12% Myristic
Milk*	69%	27%	30% Palmitic 12% Stearic 11% Myristic
Meat			
Chicken	29%	65%	42% Oleic 23% Palmitic 19% Linoleic
Turkey	30%	50%	37% Oleic 22% Palmitic 20% Linoleic
Salmon	18%	80%	25% Oleic 11% Palmitic 5% Linoleic

Lard (pig fat)	40%	65%	44% Oleic 27% Palmitic 11% Stearic
Beef fat	37%	61%	48% Oleic 27% Palmitic 11% Palmitoleic
Oils			
Coconut Oil	90%	9%	48% Lauric 16% Myristic
Olive Oil	12%	86%	78% Oleic 10% Palmitic
Corn Oil	16%	84%	52% Linoleic 31% Oleic
Palm Oil	48%	50%	44% Palmitic 40% Oleic
Peanut Oil	16%	79%	41% Linoleic 38% Oleic
Safflower Oil	10%	89%	75% Linoleic 14% Oleic
Soybean Oil	14%	81%	51% Linoleic 23% Oleic

*Milk fat contains some 400 fatty acids, making it the most "complex" natural fat.[98, 99]

Fats, Cooking, and Oxidation

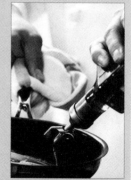

One factor to be aware of when adding fats to the diet is rancidity. This refers to the oxidation of fats, which gives off free radicals that are very harmful to the body. Just as different sources of fat have different smoke points (temperatures at which they begin breaking down), so too do these fats have different oxidative properties.

Heated and oxidized PUFAs are bad. Vegetable, nut, and seed oils contain high levels of PUFAs, which makes them unstable. They oxidize easily due to the presence of double bonds in their chemical makeup. Therefore, using these oils for cooking, frying, and deep-frying, exposes you to the detriments of oxidation.

Deep-fried, dehydrated, and powdered foods are other dietary sources of oxidized products.

What's more, dietary oxidized lipids are absorbed through the small intestine, incorporated into lipoproteins, and are released into the blood, where they can increase the risk of cardiovascular disease. It's not the LDL, but the inflamed and/or oxidized LDL that is so atherosclerotic and dangerous.[100]

Weighing In on Fats

Studies also show that high-fat diets can out-perform low-fat diets in relation to inflammatory markers[345], further demonstrating that high-fat diets are healthful, especially when it comes to inflammation.

The Best Oils for Cooking

Peanut oil is known for its high smoke point, making it one of the best cooking oils for frying. However, it has 30% omega-6, and frying causes oxidation of fatty acids, which is why we don't recommend fried foods or cooking at high temps.

Some of the oxidation dangers can be avoided by cooking with good, old-fashioned, grass-fed, beef tallow. Your great-great grandmother, who lived to 110 and died mowing the back yard, did it this way.

Saturated fats tend to be more stable, meaning that they're less likely to oxidize over time. Coconut oil, tallow, butter, and lard are all fats that are considered highly stable and not subjected to going rancid quickly. They tend to have lower smoke points, however, which is a consideration in cooking.	Because of its stability and nutritional value, **coconut oil** is what we most often use in our house and recommend to our patients. Of course, we don't fry anything, and coconut oil is not suitable for frying.
Monounsaturated fats can be used at low temperatures, but are best just added to cold, raw food, or food that's already been cooked.	**Olive oil** includes saturated fats that help keep it stable, not to mention the fact that it only has the one (mono) susceptible bond. This makes olive oil more stable than polyunsaturated fats, but it still should only be used at low temperatures, if heated at all. It shouldn't be used at high temperatures.
Polyunsaturated fats, especially those found in vegetable oil, can be a little trickier. They're the quickest to go rancid, which is especially true when they're heated; there's a reason you don't cook with fish or flax oil.	**Grape-seed oil** is considered be good for cooking because of its high smoke point. Yet, with its vulnerable chemical makeup, this fat will go rancid and oxidize as well.

To eat safe fat that hasn't gone rancid, be sure to adhere to the following tips:

- Keep fats stored at room temperature. Keeping them stored in the refrigerator will extend their life even more.
- Keep polys and monos out of the heat or sun.
- When in doubt, use fats with fewer double bonds. The fewer oxygen bonds, the less likely your fat is to have oxidized. Monounsaturated fats have fewer double bonds than polyunsaturated fats, and saturated fats have none.

Trans Fatty Acids

If there's one fat you always want to avoid, it's the fat present in trans fatty acids. Most trans fats are created through hydrogenation, the addition of extra hydrogen molecules to largely unsaturated oils, such as corn, vegetable or soybean oil.[101]

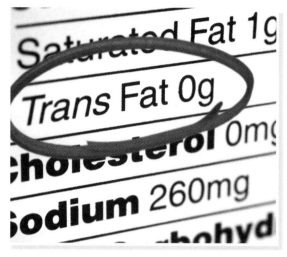

You might think of it as a "man-made" fat, and like so many other man-made foods, it's something to avoid.

Hydrogenation can move double bonds from their naturally occurring positions. After hydrogenation, the oil is termed "partially hydrogenated" (a term you're likely familiar with if you read food labels), and it contains trans fats. Here's the low-down on trans fats:

Initially created as an alternative to animal-based saturated fat sources, it turned out the alternative was much worse.

Trans Fats

Trans fatty acids are not only unessential, but actively increase your risks for a number of health problems, the most obvious of which is cardiovascular disease.

A rule of thumb: if it says "hydrogenated" or "partially-hydrogenated oil" on the back, don't eat it.

Foods: Margarine, packaged foods, cake mixes, donuts, food fried in partially-hydrogenated oil, processed baked goods, cookies, etc.

Health Comments

In a study on monkeys, trans fat was found to be a cause of weight gain known as an "independent factor." In other words, if you eat trans fats, you're more likely to put on weight.[102]

Trans fats were found to both lower HDL and raise LDL, which are associated risk factors for heart disease.[103]

Why do so many manufacturers use these hydrogenated oils in their products? Traditionally, food manufacturers mostly used natural animal fats like lard and butter when producing fried and baked goods. When scientists erroneously showed up and suggested a link between (saturated) fats and heart diseases, people wanted alternatives, and the manufacturers gave it to them.

There are a few advantages to hydrogenated oils; but all of the benefits are for the manufacturers and none are for your health. They're stable, easy to store, and they often taste good.

The problem is that the research is pretty clear on the fact that trans fats can increase LDL cholesterol as well as the risk for heart disease. But they do more than that: they also impair your ability to process omega-3 and omega-6 fatty acids properly. As you've seen, this leads to virtually any disease.[104, 105]

You can avoid these trans fats by following a few rules of thumb:

Avoid fast food and deep-fried food

Scour through nutrition labels and watch for "hydrogenated and partially hydrogenated oils."	Read labels for "trans-fats"—but realize that manufacturers can put "0 trans-fats" by reducing serving size. If the total per serving is small enough, you can still put a 0 on the score board.

The science on trans fats is in, and it's not good. Stay away from them if you want to improve your health.[106, 107, 108]

KEY CONCEPTS FROM THIS CHAPTER

1. Watch your omega-3s and omega-6s by checking their balance scores.

Go to http://www.fastlearner.org/omega3-6balance.htm to find foods rich in omega-3s that aren't "drowned out" by an unfavorable presence of omega-6s. This will help you restore your body's natural balance that prevents inflammation and obesity.

2. Saturated fats can be good for you.

There are plenty of saturated fats that come with astounding health benefits. In cooking, they're also slow to oxidize, which is why they can even be healthier than the alternative cooking oils.

3. A low-fat diet is not always a low-fat diet.

You are not what you eat, but what your body absorbs and synthesizes. Carbohydrates in the diet can convert to saturated fatty acids in the body, which is why it's important to remember that many foods are more fattening than pure fat itself.

4. Do away with the trans fats.

They're bad for you in more ways than one. While there are beneficial and essential elements of different categories of fats, there's nothing particularly beneficial or essential about trans fats. Avoiding fast, fried, and processed/baked foods will help you avoid their nasty effects.

CHAPTER SIX:

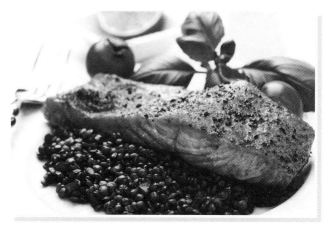

iProtein:
Create a Protein Plan
Based on You

H$_2$A$_2$ Formula Step 3

iProtein is about the personal choice you have to make to meet your protein needs. Levels and intensity of activity, age, and illness all impact how much is recommended and whether it should come from animal or plant sources.

Too little protein can lead to a number of problems and ailments, including:

Brittle hair
Weak fingernails and toenails
Muscle wasting
Low immunity
Blood disorders, such as problems clotting or with hemoglobin
Skin problems

Too much protein: Protein can be broken down into sugar, which in turn means that your body creates insulin in order to bring blood sugar levels back down to normal. This is something you look to limit in Maximized Metabolix.

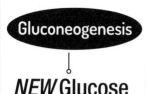

How Protein Becomes Blood Sugar

Protein can have a moderate effect on blood sugar levels through a process we've mentioned called gluconeogenesis, or "the creation of new glucose."

Glucose is not an essential nutrient in your diet because of processes like gluconeogenesis, which makes up for any glucose deficiencies. The point of mentioning this is that, while above standard recommendations, our plans are not high protein because too much protein will raise insulin and expose you to insulin's ugly parabolic, metabolic problems.

Choosing Your Protein

Depending on your activity level and health profile, you may need to switch or cut your protein. What does this mean? Switch your protein sources or cut back the percent of calories you get from protein. If you don't exercise much or you do not have access to natural, organic cows, chickens, their products, and wild, safe fish, you should cut back on the amount of animal protein in your diet.

The world famous cancer expert Dr. Charles Majors and I wrote a book called, *The Cancer Killers*. We work with cancer patients and natural cancer clinics all over the world. Most of these clinics have patients turn to vegetarianism due to the impact of unclean animal sources on the body and its immune system.

To those who choose veganism, do not have access to protein from clean animal sources, or are concerned about chronic illnesses like cancer, you can switch from animal products to plant-based proteins.

You can combine the proteins in nuts, seeds, vegetables, some legumes, and a modest amount of non-GMO, gluten-free grains throughout the day in order to get all nine essential amino acids. *(See our soaking/sprouting section in* **Appendix IX** *for notes on how to deal with plant based proteins and grains.)*

Sources of H_2A_2 Whole Food Protein

Good	Bad
Meat from whole sources like pasture-raised, 100% grass-fed beef, and free-range chicken	• Commercial feed- and grain-eating animals injected with growth hormones, steroids, and antibiotics • **Worse:** Processed meats—usually high in omega-6s and full of nitrites, which can be converted to nitrosamines, a potentially cancer-causing substance • Pork and pork products

Wild fish from the "safe fish" list	Farm-raised fish, shell fish, and other fish from the toxic list.
Dairy and eggs from whole, naturally-fed sources	Dairy products and eggs from commercially fed cows and chickens
Seeds: raw flax, hemp, pumpkin, and sunflower seeds	Large amounts of seeds—they're -3 foods, high in omega 6. Large amounts of roasted seeds.
Moderate amounts of raw walnuts, almonds, cashews	Large amounts! Avoid roasting nuts as well
Small amounts of fermented soy products	Processed and excessive soy products, i.e., soy milk, soy protein, tofu, etc.
Modest amounts of legumes: including beans, peas, and lentils (see our soaking/sprouting instructions in Appendix IX)	Large amounts are a problem due to anti-nutrients.

Good Proteins for Your Kitchen:

Safest fish, two–three times a week
Grass-fed, organic beef
Wild game
Grass-fed, organic, raw dairy
Raw butter and cheese
Pasture raised, free-range chicken and eggs
Organic turkey
Grass-fed concentrated whey protein (not isolate)

Good Protein for Vegans:

Moderate legumes: beans and lentils *(see our soaking/sprouting guide in the **Appendix IX**)*
Raw nuts and seeds *(again, see our soaking/sprouting section in the **Appendix IX** for notes on how to deal with these)*
Vegan plant protein supplement: rice, hemp, pea
Fermented soy products

Right Amount, Right Source

If you eat proteins in the right amounts—and from the right sources—you give yourself a great foundation for building muscle and losing fat.

But what, exactly, are the right amounts of "iProtein" in your diet?

Protein Quantity:
How Much Protein Should You Eat

How Much Per Meal

Conventional science puts the number at which you can absorb protein at a maximum of about 10 grams of protein per hour. Coupled with your liver's limits on its capacity to deaminate amino acids and produce urea for the excretion of excess nitrogen, you'll be able to synthesize as much as 25–30 grams per meal. You'll have to wait two to three hours for the effective metabolism of this protein before you can most efficiently take in another dose.

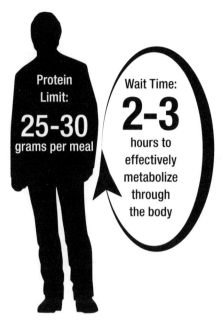

Protein Limit:

25-30 grams per meal

Wait Time:

2-3 hours to effectively metabolize through the body

There are different theories out there about the bioavailability of proteins and whether or not your body is forced to digest all of its protein over two–three hours, or whether there are longer intestinal transit times.

The bottom line? Once you hit your protein limit, the excess protein isn't helpful or healthy. The body can turn the spillover into blood sugar through a process called "gluconeogenesis." And blood sugar can turn into body fat. That's why you're better off with a smaller amount of protein divided up throughout the day rather than loading up on 50–90 grams in a single sitting.[109]

How Much Protein Per Day

The question of how much protein you should consume daily to optimize health, muscle recovery, and lean tissue preservation is important—and it's vital that you have a good answer.

Like many recommendations, the typical recommended intakes of protein tend to be "minimum daily amounts" needed for survival and avoiding diseases of deficiency. They don't give you your ideal daily amounts. They don't factor in your fitness goals, your activity levels, or other variables that make you unique from your average, or even below-average, neighbors.

The institutional dietary allowances for different age groups[110] recommends the following:

Infants (0–12 months)	Children (1–8 years)	Males and Females (9–13 years)	Males (14–18 years)	Males (19 years and over)	Females (14 years and over)
9–11 grams per day	13–19 grams per day	34 grams per day	52 grams per day	56 grams per day	46 grams per day

Note that these are not the Maximized Metabolix recommendations to thrive, but the standard "RDI" to survive.

Numerous studies have shown that diets higher in protein, above RDAs, increase overall energy expenditure by increasing the thermogenic effects of feeding as well as promoting sensation of satiety (fullness) and thus contributing to weight loss.[111]

In addition, protein diets above baseline recommendations like the ones we share, are known to have beneficial effects on body composition.[112]

On the other hand, the term "high protein" can also be a problem.

Don't Let Your Protein Get Too High

High protein diets can give you excessive amounts—amounts that overwhelm your liver's capacity to convert excess nitrogen to urea in the urine. The accepted danger zone of intake is anything greater than 35%—which will expose you to a variety of risks, some very serious.[113]

Within the range we'll be recommending of 15–25% of your calories, you'll take a hold of the advantages of protein without exposing yourself to problems of "high" protein intake.[114, 115, 116, 117]

Hard to Find?

If can't find good, organic animal meats and grass-fed organic dairy, lower the percent of your diet that is based on protein and/or minimize your use of animal proteins and use more vegetarian protein options.

When thinking about amounts per meal and per day, remember the point made earlier in this chapter: the source of your protein is also crucial. Specifically, the commercialization of animal food production has altered the biochemistry of the meat you eat—and if you don't have access to clean proteins, you'll have to rethink your protein strategies.

Choosing Your "Thrive" Protein Levels

As we look to eliminate the carbs, we're left with protein and fat as our sources of energy. A healthy (and higher than standard) amount of protein is an excellent alternative to replacing the sugars and the grains and starches that just turn into sugar anyway. If you're going to get our typical recommendation of protein at 15–25% of your calories, here's what your diet may look like:

Protein Bang For Your Calorie Buck

Calories	15%–25% of Calories	Grams
1800	270–450	68–113
2000	300–500	75–125
2400	360–600	90–150
2800	420–700	105–180 *

*Serious power athletes at five–six meals maxed out at 30–35g of protein per meal.

Vegetarians or people without access to or the finances to eat quality protein products should or will lean more to the 15% side. Those that are very physically active, athletes, bodybuilders, etc., are going to lean more to that 25+% side.

Within the ranges suggested of 15–25%, there's nothing to support risk of kidney function or the other suggested protein issues like osteoporosis, cancer, dehydration, colon, or liver problems.[118, 119, 120, 121] To get the right protein levels, just get your 20–30g per meal until you hit your mark.

Example Protein Choices to Hit Your Mark

See also the Protein Counter in Chapter Seven. There you'll find a chart full of examples of foods that will give you 20–30 grams of protein. You'll also find a guide there that displays how much protein you can expect out of common, whole, protein-rich foods.

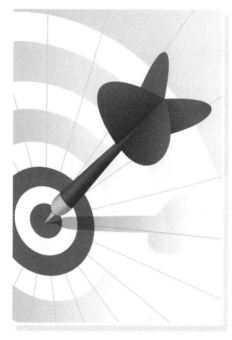

Four eggs (24g) with cheese (6g)	**30g**
Protein shake with grass-fed whey (25g) and chia seeds (4g)	**29g**
Lunch of 5 oz. salmon (30g) salad with ground flax seeds (8g)	**38g**
Snack of cashews (5g) and almonds (7g)	**12g**
Dinner—chicken (3oz)	**32g**
Total protein	**141g**

Is Protein Harmful to Your Kidneys?

A simple process happens when you burn protein as fuel: This isn't a bad side-effect of eating

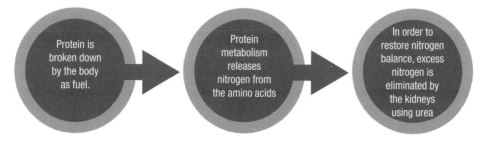

Protein is broken down by the body as fuel. → Protein metabolism releases nitrogen from the amino acids → In order to restore nitrogen balance, excess nitrogen is eliminated by the kidneys using urea

protein; it's how your body should work. The idea that protein causes kidney damage arises from this basic sequence of events.

The truth is that some people with a pre-existing kidney disease can have trouble with eating too much protein. But if your kidneys are already working just fine, then a moderate increase in protein shouldn't blow out your kidneys.

Although the research is still inconclusive, a review of the issue published in *Nutrition & Metabolism*[122] found that "Although excessive protein intake remains a health concern in individuals with pre-existing renal disease, the literature lacks significant research demonstrating a link between protein intake and the initiation or progression of renal disease in healthy individuals."

Metabolix eating is not "high protein." But if your kidneys already work, you shouldn't need to worry, anyway.

Protein for Athletes

We'll touch more on protein for athletes in Appendix VII, on Fitness and Exercise. For now, know that by adding a 20–30g protein meal after a workout and adding one–two other small protein meals per day, you can easily meet your protein needs.[123]

Protein Quality:
The Health Benefits of Treating Animals Well

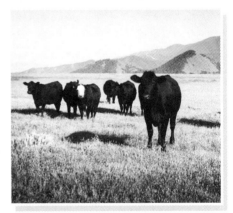

It shouldn't come as a surprise that the better fed our meat has been, the better the meat itself will be. But what exactly defines "better fed" depends upon the animal itself—as do the health benefits you can see by finding more natural sources of meat that come from animals who have been fed well.

Grass-fed and finished beef produces leaner cows as well as a better fat profile in the meat. Pastured beef is higher in omega-3 fatty acids and lower in omega-6 than grain-fed counterparts, which is extremely important to your health. It's worth noting that even the cheese produced by grass-fed cows is higher in nutritional elements like CLA than the cheese from grain-fed cows.

Grass-finished is important. Meat producers can still call their cattle "grass-fed," yet finish with grains and still end up changing the quality of the meat and the fatty acid content.

Natural Grass-fed Cows vs. Commercial, Grain-Fed Cows

Higher in vitamin E[124]

Higher in B-vitamins thiamin and riboflavin[124]

Higher in total omega-3s[125]

Higher in CLA[126]

Higher in beta-carotene[127]

More anti-oxidants, more CLA, more calcium, magnesium and potassium[124]

Vastly superior omega-3 to omega-6 ratio[124]

Better Fed, Better Benefits

Pastured beef is higher in omega-3 fatty acids and lower in omega-6 than grain-fed counterparts, which is extremely important to your health.

Cheese

Cheese from grass-fed sources not only has a much improved omega-6 to omega-3 ratio, but offers higher amounts of calcium, magnesium, and vitamins A, C, D, and E. Hard cheese like Parmesan pack a lot of the protein power of milk without as much of the lactose.

Many people associate the problems of cheese with highly processed foods, but "real" cheese is simple: it's essentially milk and enzymes. It's when the other "stuff" is added, allowing you to eat cheese from a can, that the problems start to add up. Find the real stuff: Gouda, Brie, Cheddar, Gruyere, Parmesan, etc.

Free-range chickens or "pastured" chickens are exactly what they sound like—chickens that have been freed to roam about a yard, giving them access to natural food sources like insects while allowing them to exercise.

One problem is that free-range eggs do not have a standard definition in the United States, so you may want to research more about your local food sources. Your free-range chickens might not really be "free" and still eat the grain their farmers are feeding them.

TOXIC EFFECTS

Food producers, product manufacturers, government officials, pharmaceutical companies, medical professionals and others will admit that while the chemicals present in products could be harmful in high doses, they're perfectly safe in the small amounts that a product contains.

If we are exposed only once in our lives, that might be a meaningful statement. The problem is we are exposed repeatedly to these chemicals. Over time, they build up in our systems.

While you are not likely to get cancer from one injection at your pediatrician's office; one diet cola, one cigarette, one order of fast food, a new-car smell, or a couple of pieces of pizza, these toxic materials can't be effectively metabolized by your body.

These toxins, and the physiological impact they make and build up in your system, create what is called a "toxic burden." This gradual physiological decline, and the buildup in your blood, cells, tissues, or organs can be undetectable for years, until symptoms start to become obvious. Over time, the burden becomes too great for the body to carry.

Free-range chickens are:

Higher in folate	*Higher in beta carotene*
Higher in omega-3s	*Higher in vitamins A, D, E, and B12.*

… than their commercial counter parts. Free-range eggs are better, too. They have more beta-carotene, vitamin A, and more omega-3 fatty acids. In fact, there were 100% more omega-3s in the free-range eggs.[128]

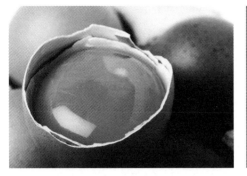

Eat the Yolk

Many people avoid egg yolks because of the cholesterol content, forgetting all of the nutrition present: vitamin D, vitamin A, choline, and more! If you want to harness the full nutritive power of the egg, eat the yolk!

The egg's reputation over the years has been somewhat tarnished thanks to a high amount of cholesterol in the yolks. Yet, as we covered, we've known for years that dietary cholesterol has little to do with serum (blood) cholesterol.

If it's a commercially produced, non-free-range egg, you'd want to limit some of the yolks due to poorer, negative concentrations of omega 3—not to mention toxicity.

With good eggs, however, if you eat egg whites only, you'll also lose rich nutrients like choline, vitamin D, vitamin A, vitamin B-12, and others.

Wild Fish

Wild fish are much better than farm-raised fish. Fish advertised as "Alaskan salmon" is often raised on a fish farm where they're fed with things that fish aren't meant to eat. Unfortunately, farmed fish represent a majority of the salmon market today.

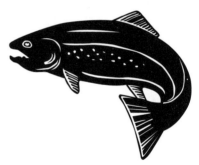

Wild fish:

Higher in omega-3 fatty acids
Improved omega-3 to omega-6 ratio
Have far fewer polychlorinated biphenyls than farm-raised salmon. These chemicals have been linked to cancer.[129]

A serious concern when eating fish is to be sure that you're avoiding high levels of mercury. Here's a quick guide to ensuring that you eat the right fish:

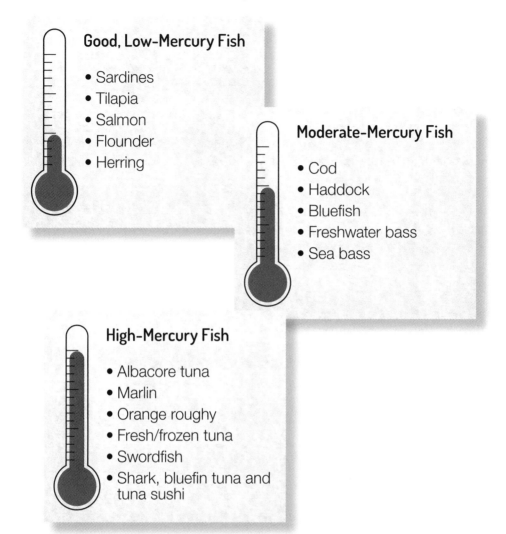

Good, Low-Mercury Fish

- Sardines
- Tilapia
- Salmon
- Flounder
- Herring

Moderate-Mercury Fish

- Cod
- Haddock
- Bluefish
- Freshwater bass
- Sea bass

High-Mercury Fish

- Albacore tuna
- Marlin
- Orange roughy
- Fresh/frozen tuna
- Swordfish
- Shark, bluefin tuna and tuna sushi

Toxic Bottom Feeders

Crab, lobster, mussels, oysters, scallops, and shrimp are bottom-feeding scavengers. Since your food is made up of what it eats, you want to dramatically limit your intake of these toxin-containing seafoods.

Dairy:
Are Milk and Milk Products Good for You?

As with the beef, the milk of the cow has a whole lot to do with how it's raised and what you feed it. Commercial dairy products, where the cows were raised on grains and injected with hormones and other drugs, is definitely not recommended as part of anyone's regular diet—no matter what you've heard or read in a "Got Milk?" ad.

Some people may be sensitive to milk and dairy products. But, to understand dairy, you have to understand two things: the source of the milk and the proteins it contains.

Where does it come from? Like you saw with the meat from cows, the milk from cows has much higher omega-3 levels, a far better omega-6:3 ratio, and greater levels of CLA and other good nutrients.

Data connecting dairy products to heart disease and cancer do not consider pasture-raised vs. commercially-raised cows, and have either been highly inconclusive or shown no link at all.

Lose the Soy Milk

Nearly all soy protein comes from GMO (genetically modified organisms) soybeans. In order to turn them into milk, they have to be processed at high heat. If not, the dangerous phytic acid levels are too high and can cause harm by blocking essential nutrients from being absorbed in your body.

Other milks like rice or almond milk don't carry the dangers of soy. Yet they're still highly processed unless you've made them at home.

The research that does show problems is likely done using commercial dairy products only. There are studies that reveal that nonorganic cow's milk produced from cows treated with rBGH (growth hormones) increases the risk for breast cancer and colon cancer. Nonorganic milk found on store shelves contains rBGH and other synthetics, which are known hormone disruptors. They can, for example, lead to circulating concentrations of insulin-like growth factor-1, thus potentially increasing the risk of breast cancer.[130, 131, 132]

What are the proteins in the milk? The two proteins in milk are:

- ## Casein is the most common
- ## Lactalbumin or whey

Casein, along with the lactose sugar, is the compound that most people are allergic or intolerant of.

The first thing you want to look for with dairy is that it comes from pasture-raised, grass-fed and finished cows that are organic—not given antibiotics, hormones, and other drugs. You'll often find that there is not the sensitivity to proteins and lactose in dairy that has been raised properly.

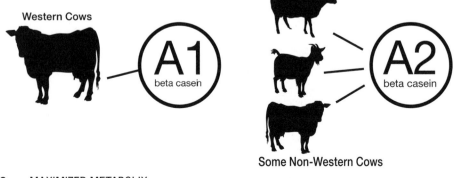

Western Cows

A1 beta casein

Some Non-Western Cows

A2 beta casein

There are two types of casein: A1 and A2 beta casein. It's been hypothesized that the A1, common in western dairy cows, is the reason so many people are intolerant of dairy products. Goat, sheep, and buffalo milk are A2 casein and most people can tolerate their dairy products.

Many people also respond poorly to commercial, refined whey protein. On the contrary, the high quality, grass-fed whey protein we recommend in the supplement **Chapter Seven** of the book is casein- and lactose-free to reduce milk protein and sugar sensitivities.

Dairy and Heart Disease

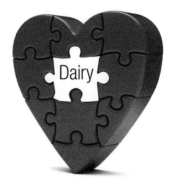

Recently, moderate evidence also suggests that intake of milk and milk products are associated with a reduced risk of cardiovascular disease and type 2 diabetes in adults.[133]

While tradition has been to condemn dairy products based on their saturated fat levels and their involvement in heart disease, the actual evidence has not shown that higher intakes of milk and dairy products, regardless of milk fat levels, are associated with an increased risk of CVD, coronary heart disease (CHD), or stroke.[134, 135, 136, 137]

In fact, in one carefully designed analysis—of many studies that examined different dairy food categories and different ranges of intake—, showed a modest inverse association between milk intake and overall CVD risk (i.e., CHD and stroke). Specifically, milk intake was found not to be associated with the risk of CHD, total mortality, or stroke.[138]

As far as *high-fat vs. low-fat* dairy—there is limited information on the specific influence of high-fat and lower fat dairy consumption and heart disease risk. In general, those studies that examined the association between the intake of total high-fat or total low-fat dairy products and the risk of CHD or stroke, many reported no associations. .[139]

Consequently, until there is consensus, these results suggest caution only when recommending whole-milk consumption for those at the greatest risk of CHD and stroke.

On the topic of milk fats and cholesterol, while there is evidence of a rise in LDL, there's also a rise in the good HDL.[140, 141, 142]

That said, dairy is not nature's perfect food for adults. In the case of commercial, grain- and hormone- fed cows, it appears advisable on many levels to significantly reduce, or better yet, avoid completely. On the other hand, making the right, tolerable, amount of naturally raised dairy products a moderate part of your diet hasn't been shown to be of any great concern and can provide many benefits.

Protein Supplementation:
Is It Right for You?

To increase protein to desired levels, many people require a supplement. This is particularly true of athletes and others who train regularly. Whey from milk has been found to be a great biologically available supplement source. But, like any animal product—particularly dairy—where the protein comes from and how the animals were treated plays a huge role as to whether or not it will be healthy.

See more about grass-fed whey in the Supplement **Chapter Seven**.

In obese subjects, consumption of a diet enriched in milk-whey protein (a by-product of cheese production) led to significant weight loss and smaller waist circumference compared with subjects supplemented with soy protein.[143]

Whey protein is also believed to increase energy expenditure, suppress appetite, aid in detoxification, and promote weight loss. Whey proteins are rich in leucine, and an excellent source of energy and new protein for skeletal muscle.

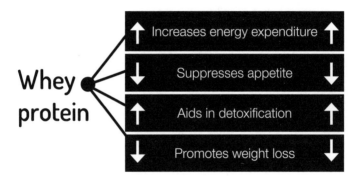

If you're not sure this is right for you, consider that a 2008 paper[144] concluded that protein can help you regulate your body weight through three factors:

> **Retaining lean mass while still allowing fat loss**
>
> **Increasing satiety, or feelings of fullness. This allows you to consume fewer calories naturally**
>
> **Helping you to regain less weight after a diet**

What are we to conclude? If you want to maintain lean mass and reduce the fat in your body, at least a moderate intake of protein will not only be beneficial, but necessary. This is particularly important when following our recommendations for lower-carb eating.

Getting Protein
as a Vegetarian

Is it true that complementary proteins must be eaten together to count as a protein source?

In the past, it was thought that these complementary proteins needed to be eaten at the same meal for your body to use them together. Now studies show that your body can combine complementary proteins that are eaten within the same day.[145]

For meat-eaters, getting enough of protein's nine essential amino acids is not difficult. Eggs, many meats, and even dairy products are known to be "complete" sources of protein—when eaten regularly enough, they keep your body fueled with enough protein to get by just fine.

For vegetarians, getting protein is a little trickier. Vegetarians that allow themselves some animal products, like eggs and dairy, have access to complete proteins that are rich in essential amino acids like methionine and cysteine.

For vegans—who forgo animal products entirely—soy is often relied on to get an adequate intake of protein. Soy was once lauded as a cholesterol-lowering, heart-healthy food, but recent research suggests that it's not so innocent. As it turns out, the soybean has a somewhat questionable record when it comes to health and wellness.

Consider some of the evidence:

A 2008 study in the Journal of Nutrition found that "Overall, existing data are inconsistent or inadequate in supporting most of the suggested health benefits of consuming soy protein or ISF." ISF stands for isoflavones, a group of organic compounds that can be found in soy.[146]

A review published in 2007[147] noted that "it does not seem that soy and its constituent isoflavones have met original expectations."

Despite soy's reputation as a heart-healthy protein, a 2006 study in Circulation found only a minimal effect of soy consumption on cholesterol levels.[148]

A review published in Circulation found[149] "Earlier research indicating that soy protein, as compared with other proteins, has clinically important favorable effects on LDL cholesterol and other CVD risk factors has not been confirmed by many studies reported during the past 10 years." Eventually the American Heart Association made a point not to recommend isoflavone supplements.

These studies call into question the health benefits of soy—but some evidence has actively questioned whether soy might have negative effects on your health. Consider:

Soy is high in phytic acid. The problem here is that phytic acid can block your digestive system's absorption of minerals.

Soy is a phytoestrogen, which means it has an impact on the estrogen levels in your body. This is a concern for children, men, and women alike, as throwing your hormones out of balance can have adverse consequences.

Soy also contains trypsin inhibitors. Since trypsin is a digestive enzyme made in your pancreas, it's no wonder that some people have problems digesting soy, leading to diarrhea, gas, and bloating.

In animal studies, the phytoestrogens present in soy have lowered testosterone levels. In human males, eating soy may even lead to decreased sperm count.[150]

Soy has also been associated with thyroid problems, getting categorized as a "goitrogen," or a food that can promote the formation of a goiter (enlarged thyroid). If you have thyroid issues, you may want to talk to your doctor about your soy intake.

It's worth noting that, like grains, soybeans require processing before they're fit for human consumption. Fermented soy products, which often appear in the healthier Asian cultures, represent healthier sources of soy in the diet.

Yes, it is possible to get adequate protein on a diet completely devoid of animal products. But it will require a little more work, making sure that the proteins come from adequate, whole sources rather than processed products like soy.

Plant Protein Supplements

For those that are lactose-intolerant or vegan, sprouted, gluten-free grains, seeds, and legumes can replace whey. The sprouting reduces the impact of anti-nutrients that exist in grains.

To be both good for you and truly vegetarian, a plant-based protein supplement should be free of dairy, soy, gluten, or artificial flavors, artificial sweeteners, or preservatives.
See the **Chapter Seven** for recommendations.

KEY CONCEPTS FROM THIS CHAPTER

1. Your body can only handle so much protein at once.

Don't overload it; you don't want excess energy from protein. Instead, pay careful attention to the recommendations in this chapter to find your ideal protein requirements. Use the food guides to see which foods can get you the efficient, complete proteins you need throughout the day in order to get as much protein as you need— and no more. You don't want too much protein to convert to excess energy.

2. Whole food means meat that was treated well.

Pasture-raised, free-range, 100% grass-fed—these are the key phrases that will unlock an entirely new nutritional world for you. Naturally-raised, well-fed animals offer meat with more vitamins, more omega-3s, more beta-carotene. In short, if your meat is treated well, it will treat you well.

3. You can combine proteins throughout the day.

If you're a low meat eater or even a vegetarian, you can still get complete proteins throughout the day by combining various foods. As long as you do this throughout the day, you shouldn't have any problems—it's not necessary that you do it at every meal.

4. Soy is not the ideal protein you once thought it was.

It has too many negative effects! It's a good plant source of protein, sure, but beyond that, it's best to get your protein from other whole sources like the sources you read about in this chapter.

CHAPTER SEVEN:

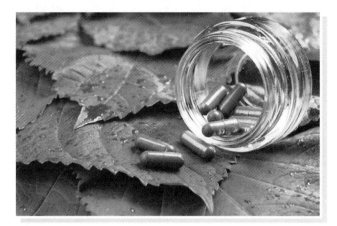

Maximized Supplementation

The Curious Case of the World of Supplements

Your body's health is not based solely on calories and the numbers of carbs you eat. It depends on the nutrients you actually absorb. This is easily missed in many programs that just focus on your weight.

It's a common thought that if you eat well then you don't need to take a supplement. Of course, the first question should be, "Are you really eating that well?" Ultimately, we all need a supplement plan.

A Supplement is Exactly That:

It's meant to *supplement* good nutrition

What we know today is that it's very unlikely—and perhaps impossible—to really get all of the micronutrients you need from diet. And this is likely the case even if you're eating all your fruits and vegetables.

Modern, commercial food production has promoted the push for fast-paced agricultural practices. This includes the use of chemicals, genetically modified organisms (GMOs), and other processes done for ease, profit, and expediency. Yes—we have larger yields of foods, but at what cost? All these practices are ultimately stripping the soil of nutrients and causing troubling health implications, both physical and mental. Today, you would need to eat five oranges to get the same amount of vitamin A your grandparents would have gotten from one.[151]

A landmark study on the topic by Donald Davis and his team of researchers from the University of Texas at Austin's Department of Chemistry and Biochemistry was published in *December 2004 in the Journal of the American College of Nutrition*. They studied US Department of Agriculture nutritional data from both 1950 and 1999 for forty-three different vegetables and fruits, finding "reliable declines" in the amount of protein, calcium, phosphorus, iron, riboflavin (vitamin B2) and vitamin C over the past half-century.

Another analysis from the Kushi Institute looked at nutrient data from 1975 to 1997. They found that average calcium levels in twelve fresh vegetables dropped twenty-seven percent; iron levels, thirty-seven percent; vitamin A levels, twenty-one percent; and vitamin C levels, thirty percent.

What About What You Absorb?

Due to modern living, a mass preponderance of people now experience some form of digestive imbalance, like heartburn, bloating, diarrhea or constipation. Resultantly, even if you're taking in the nutrients, you may not actually be absorbing them.

This leaves us not only as being nutrient deficient due to poor food quality, but also facing the double whammy of **reduced absorption** of what little nutrients are there.

Because our vitamins and minerals are the co-factors involved in hundreds of energy-producing reactions, hormone systems, and free-radical protection, we must supplement our diets with high quality nutrients that are readily absorbable or risk increasing our chances of many chronic diseases, including cardiovascular disease, diabetes, obesity, Alzheimer's or dementia, and cancer.

Heart conditions, for example, have been linked to deficiencies in copper, magnesium, potassium, and selenium, while asthma has been linked to magnesium deficiency.

A longevity study run by a team at the University of McMaster, showed that by using a cocktail of thirty-one of the most common supplements that have been researched to be beneficial for maintaining optimal brain function and mobility, the test group of mice lived longer with a higher quality of life in a more youthful state.[152] However, there are not many people who can take over thirty-one different supplements each day, so how do you know which supplements are the most important for you?

Getting Eaten Alive by the Trillion-Dollar Supplement Industry

While it's clear you need to supplement, where do you go when you're getting hit by literally millions of good, bad, and snake-oil pill, powder, and potion ads a day? In truth, if you want to get actual results and not just spend money, you need both quality products and a plan targeted to meet actual human needs.

It has been said that vitamins give you expensive urine. While that's categorically wrong in general, for millions of people it's absolutely true. We tell many of our patients that they should just flush their entire cabinet full of cheap supplements down the toilet and cut out the middle man. In many cases, you would be better off—and far less toxic—eating tiny rocks.

Your body, and the nutrients that it needs to be in optimal health, is as unique as your personality. Additionally, the quality you need in a vitamin is no different than the quality you need in a steak or an apple. You wouldn't (hopefully) eat a steak from a dog or cat or eat a rotten apple—just like you shouldn't take just any synthetic supplement you find for three dollars at a discount pharmacy or department store.

Choosing the Right Plan

There are essentially three paths people take when supplementing.

1. The random, inconsistent plan. This common path contains a medicine cabinet or cupboard filled with various products of differing qualities for different purposes with several having gone past their expiration dates.	BENEFITS: None
	CONCERNS: This approach is obviously not effective. What's most disconcerting is that the cheap, synthetic supplements and miracle pills that often fill these cabinets can be toxic and/or actually create health problems.
2. A personalized plan. A metabolic assessment of your health that analyzes biomarkers found in your urine and blood can tell you specifically what your personal needs are to supplement and address.	BENEFITS: These biomarkers act as a "window" to your health and indicate diseases that may be emerging. This gives you the ability to be proactive (vs. reactive) when it comes to a supplement plan and creates a future of true maximized living.
	CONCERNS: None
3. The whole food, wellness plan. Utilize quality supplements that meet the common nutritional requirements that the average person has. This approach acknowledges that most people have a need to supplement vitamin D, omegas, require a multi-vitamin, have to address regular exposure to toxins, and several others common factors.	BENEFITS: If key areas are addressed consistently, this path is likely helpful to very helpful.
	CONCERNS: Unique needs and deficiencies are not investigated, which can leave the person vulnerable to problems related to insufficient nutrients and the resulting presence or development of symptoms and illness. This is best as a follow up to #2.

As a doctor who loves people and has dealt with hundreds of thousands of patients over twenty-five years, this second pathway of testing is obviously my favorite. For my family and friends, I want to know exactly what is going on, so I can determine the most efficient, most cost-effective, and overall best approach. Personally, I want to take the fewest supplements necessary but not miss anything my body absolutely needs to thrive and feel good.

What is Biomarker Testing?

Science has discovered a way to look at biomarkers in the urine and blood to determine nutritional needs based on how various essential systems in your body are working. Lab testing for biomarkers is very important to illuminate, like a flashlight, to show where you are and where you need to go.

A customized metabolic assessment will look at different key biomarkers, which are indicative of overall health. These kinds of tests will look at markers like vitamin deficiencies, inflammation, oxidative stress, toxicity, gastrointestinal stress, stress hormone imbalance, and fatty acid imbalance. These are all areas we've touched on in this book and are common areas of metabolic maladies.

A Word of Caution

When it comes to choosing what products to take, self-diagnosis can be a damaging and even dangerous habit. Supplements and the corresponding dosages should be recommended by an expert. Browsing the aisles of the local drug stores for supplements that haven't been recommended or evaluated by your doctor can yield poor results.

For Example:

It is true, that over a fifty-year period, the average content of calcium in vegetables has declined eighty-one percent from the original levels.[153] Commonly, older women suffer from calcium deficiency. One woman who knows these facts may attempt to supplement her diet with a high-dosage of calcium. This can cause a toxic build-up that yields painful side effects, like constipation and kidney stones. Plus, this generic dosage does not target her individual needs.

The deficiency may stem from a lack of calcium in the individual's diet, or, if the diet contains adequate calcium, a digestive issue may be preventing the body from absorbing the mineral. Also, calcium is a competitive mineral that can inhibit the body's ability to absorb other vital nutrients like zinc, iron, manganese and other minerals, which could yield different problems altogether.

Finally, vitamin D is known to boost the body's ability to absorb and utilize calcium. Therefore, if sufficient calcium is available in an individual's diet, then maybe the real solution is to supplement with vitamin D.

The above example is meant to illustrate the potential complexities of beginning a supplementation program. Specific testing, administered by a qualified doctor or health care professional, should be utilized to determine individual supplementation needs.

The goal is to integrate the lab results and protocols in two phases; **Phase I:** The Therapeutic Phase, where higher doses of supplements are used to restore and saturate the tissues with depleted nutrients, and **Phase II:** The Maintenance Phase, where the cells will continually be supplied the optimal doses of longevity promoting nutrients—but with a more targeted understanding of what you personally need.

An additional, and even vital, benefit to getting tested is that often, many people find they have deficiencies they must "treat" with a higher, long-term dose during the maintenance phase (like magnesium or B12).

Choosing The Right Supplements

Whole foods have a greater level of bioavailability than foods that have been heavily processed. Bioavailability refers to a nutrient's ability to be both absorbed and utilized by your body. When you look at a food label, while there are many nutrients listed, only a fraction of them can really be absorbed by the body. The nutrients that are of poor quality and not bioavailable simply pass right through the body or worse, linger in the form of toxins.

The same is true of supplements. Whole-food supplements maximize the ability of your body to absorb and utilize the nutrients. On the other hand, cheap synthetic versions generally pass right through—or even create toxicities.

Clinical Supplements
The Therapeutic Dose

The exceptions to the synthetic rule are high quality brands of vitamins, scientifically designed to provide a pharmacological dose necessary to correct significant vitamin deficiencies as determined by testing.

Whole-foods vitamins, minerals, proteins, fats, enzymes, etc., offer nutrients in their natural form. They are easier on the digestive system because they contain all of the nutrients, co-nutrients, and co-factors synergistically necessary for the important elements to be actually assimilated by the body.

Use caution in your purchases. A recent study, conducted by the Government Accountability Office, reviewed the makeup of forty different herbal supplements.[154] Thirty-seven of the products reviewed were determined to contain various amounts of lead, mercury, arsenic, and other dangerous substances. That's a 92.5 percent rate of failure. Needless to say, picking a quality supplement from a drug store shelf is likely to turn out poorly.

Corrective Supplementation

There are a handful of powerful supplements that can be used to overcome acute issues. These are the common clinical formulas our doctors recommend:

CoQ10 and Lipoic Acid

CoQ10 is essential for the health of all human tissues and organs. Drugs that reduce cholesterol also reduce CoQ10, which makes it vitally important for anyone using statin drugs to supplement CoQ10. Lipoic acid is crucial because it is a "universal antioxidant." It is able to neutralize free radicals everywhere in the body. It can also strengthen other antioxidants (like vitamins C and E) and can even regenerate glutathione.

B-Complex

B vitamins are necessary for energy and for the function of your blood, hormones and nervous system. Because they are water-soluble and are not stored in the body (with the exception of vitamin B12), we must consume them daily. L-methylfolate is necessary because it is the naturally occurring form of folate found in cells and is more readily absorbed and utilized by the body.

Magnesium

More than 300 biochemical reactions within the human body require magnesium, including the citric acid cycle, which produces energy, bowel regulation, bone health, muscle function, kidney function, heart function. and blood pressure. This is an extremely common deficiency.

L-Glutamine

This amino acid is vital for healthy immune function and energy. It is one of the most effective supplements for healing the digestive tract (Crohn's disease, ulcerative colitis, etc.).

L-Carnitine

L-carnitine helps the body produce energy. It is important for heart and brain function, muscle movement, and many other body processes. Carnitine transports fatty acids inside the mitochondria for utilization to produce energy with vitamin B2.

Highly Concentrated Fish Oil

Advanced omega-3 research suggests benefits like improved cardiovascular health, cognitive function, immune system, and mood; but the generic omega supplements have been processed excessively and overheated. The best omega supplement will have been treated at relatively low heat and subjected to third-party testing to ensure low levels of oxidation and undetectable levels of dioxins, pesticides and heavy metals like mercury.

5-HTP

5-HTP is a precursor of serotonin. Serotonin is an important neurotransmitter which is vital to the regulation of appetite, mood, and melatonin production. The presence of serotonin in the brain is associated with a balanced emotional state. Vitamin B6 is required for the conversion of 5-HTP to serotonin. 5-HTP from the griffonia plant is more effective than tryptophan—which is made synthetically or through bacterial fermentation—because it is more readily utilized by the body.

Stress Hormone Balancer (Calming)

This type of supplement assists with muscle and nerve function, while also helping the liver process fats. Ideally, it should provide gamma-aminobutyric acid (GABA), a neurotransmitter crucial to pituitary health that regulates growth hormone production, body temperature, and also improves sleep cycles. It should also contain the non-essential amino acid glycine, which can help boost certain neurotransmitters to relax the body and reduce anxiety.

Stress Hormone Balancer (Stimulating)

This type of supplement stimulates the brain by supporting the production of the neurotransmitter dopamine, and the hormones norepinephrine and epinephrine (adrenaline). Increased dopamine improves concentration, movement, emotional response, attention, and focus. Look for one that contains an adaptogen (a natural stress reliever) called rhodiola rosea that improves resistance to biological and chemical stresses. Ideally, this type of supplement will also feature the essential amino acid methionine and octacosanol, a compound typically found in healthy vegetable oils. Combined, these ingredients provide additional synergistic support for the brain.

Free-form amino acids

Free-form amino acids are single amino acids, which need no digestion. Free-form amino acids can create enzymes, hormones, muscle tissue, and nervous tissue whenever and wherever your body needs them.

Supplementation Necessary
for Long-Term Health

Once acute issues have been resolved, maintaining a healthy system becomes the new primary goal. Maintenance supplementation is an essential portion of ensuring previous health issues never return.

Research has identified a handful of supplement types that are vital to ongoing, lifelong health. A long-term deficiency in any of the following areas can lead to serious illness, making maintenance care absolutely critical to lifelong well-being.

Natural Multivitamin

Decades of over-farming and genetic modification of food have depleted the nutrient content of our food supply. A multivitamin derived from organic, whole foods will ensure you are consuming the natural forms of vitamins and minerals lacking in the modern food supply.

Vitamin D3

High-quality vitamin D3 supports health in countless ways. From boosting heart and bone health to and lessening inflammation and the risks of certain diseases, vitamin D is vital to ongoing health.[155] Vitamin D-deficiency, on the other hand, increases risk of stroke and heart failure.[156, 157] While the human body produces vitamin D naturally when exposed to moderate sunlight, indoor jobs and cold weather climates have left nearly half of all Americans vitamin D-deficient.[158]

Senior author Bess Dawson-Hughes, M.D., director of the Bone Metabolism Laboratory at the Jean Mayer USDA Human Nutrition and Research Center on Aging at Tufts University, says, "We may need to reconsider the current recommended daily values of vitamin D for older adults." Dawson-Hughes believes that "vitamin D may also improve muscle strength, thereby reducing fracture risk through fall prevention."[159]

Emerging science suggests that vitamin D receptors are found throughout the body. Over 900 genes and several areas of the body have vitamin D receptors, or proteins that bind to vitamin D.[160] According to University of California Riverside's Biochemistry Presidential Chair, this means that, "vitamin D supports immune system, pancreas, heart, blood, cellular, muscle, bone and bone marrow, breast, colon, intestine, kidney, lung, prostate, retina, skin, stomach, uterine, and brain health—and can [positively] impact thirty-six bodily organs." Even improved memory and concentration have been linked to vitamin D intake![161]

Vitamin D can also inhibit unwanted and unhealthy cell proliferation, while stimulating healthy cell differentiation.[162] When some cells divide rapidly, or proliferate, the impact on your health can be devastating. Cell differentiation, however, can decrease unwanted cellular proliferation. Lung, skin, colon, bone and breast sites have been studied for vitamin D's positive effects on cell proliferation and differentiation. Vitamin D causes cells to act as normal, mature cells by stimulating healthy cell differentiation. Dr. Cedric Garland, a twenty-year veteran vitamin D researcher, believes vitamin D can prevent unwanted cell proliferation by seventy percent with optimal vitamin D blood levels.[163]

Many vitamin D supplement options are available, but nearly all contain synthetic versions derived from irradiated animal fat.[164] A whole-foods option would provide the needed amount of vitamin D3 without a risk of excess sun exposure.

Clean Whey Protein

Quality protein comprises the building blocks of a healthy body by repairing muscles and bones, providing a source of energy, and boosting your metabolism. Whey protein is nature's richest source of biologically-available protein, complete with all twenty-two essential amino acids. Whey protein contains powerful immune boosters and helps to synthesize antioxidants necessary for detoxification. Studies by Dr. Donald Layman, a professor at the University of Illinois, have highlighted the role of the essential amino acid leucine in improving body composition.[165] High quality whey protein is rich in leucine to help preserve lean muscle tissue while promoting fat loss. Research out of the International Journal of Food Sciences and Nutrition suggests that whey protein can increase cellular levels of glutathione—an antioxidant that defends the body against free radical damage, toxins, and cancer.[166]

Whey protein also helps stabilize blood glucose levels by slowing the absorption of glucose into the bloodstream. This in turn reduces hunger by lowering insulin levels and making it easier for the body to burn fat.[167]

The best sources of whey protein will be derived from one hundred-percent naturally-raised cows that have never been injected with hormones and were allowed to graze on natural grass pastures free of pesticides and chemicals. Additionally, the protein should have been subjected to low-temperature delicate filtration to protect its vital enzymes, immune factors, amino acids and overall nutrient content.

Plant-based Protein

For those who are vegan, vegetarian or lactose intolerant, a plant-based protein powder derived from whole vegetables can provide strong antioxidant benefits as well as help improve body composition. A quality source of plant protein will feature low-glycemic brown rice protein, less than one gram of sugar, and be verified as one hundred-percent soy-free (soy is one of the world's most notorious genetically modified crops). The ideal blend will feature an extensive blend of seeds and sprouts.

Natural Anti-inflammatory

Busy lives and nutrient-poor diets cause oxidative stress and inflammation. An anti-inflammatory supplement will support the body's natural defense mechanisms against free radical damage and inflammation, down to the cellular level. The ideal supplement will contain naturally soothing ingredients like turmeric and amla berry.[168, 169] Over-the-counter pain relievers may reduce pain in the short-term, but their synthetic makeup leaves a chemical trail that is toxic to the body. [170]

Cellular Detoxification Agent

No matter where we live, work or play, we are always exposed to some level of toxins that are harmful to the human body. Inevitably, these environmental toxins infiltrate the bloodstream via foods, beverages, medications and even the air.[171] Even the healthiest of people absorb toxins on a regular basis. If left unaddressed, these toxins can accumulate in the body cause the development of disease.[172] The human body must battle daily to remove dangerous chemicals, parasites and heavy metals from its cells. This detoxification process must be supported with a special formulation that can escort these toxins out of the bloodstream first, and then out of the body entirely. Look for supplements containing natural detoxification ingredients like chlorella, milk thistle, and activated charcoal. The most effective detox supplements will also provide the building blocks needed to produce the body's most powerful antioxidant, glutathione.

Greens

Green vegetables provide the nutrients needed to ensure proper digestion and allow the body to age slowly and naturally.[173, 174] The standard North American diet is grossly lacking in vegetables, which necessitates ongoing greens supplementation. An exceptional greens supplement will contain a blend of raw vegetables and live grass juices. Raw supplements are loaded with essential nutrients that the body needs in order to properly absorb vitamins and minerals. Using a raw supplement is also a more natural form of nutrients that the body recognizes. These raw veggies should include a wide variety of whole vegetable to maximize their cumulative antioxidant, anti-inflammatory impact. Kale, beets, carrots, sprouts, and more should be included.

Omega 3 and 6

Omega fatty acids Omega-3s are some of the good fats that are critical to a healthy diet, but they are not naturally produced in your body. Thus, they must be continually consumed from external sources in order to experience the improvement in mood, immune function, joint mobility, and decreases inflammation.[175, 176, 177, 178] The ideal omega supplement will provide an appropriate ratio (2:1–4:1) of omega-6 to omega-3 fatty acids, and the omegas themselves should be derived from natural sources, like fish oil and flaxseed oil.[179] If possible, choose a supplement that also contains significant amounts of gamma-linolenic acid. Commonly referred to as GLA, this substance can help improve skin health, relieve symptoms of rheumatoid arthritis and even counteract the nutrition imbalances associated with asthma, allergies and atherosclerosis.[180]

Gut Repair and Digestive Health

The standard North American diet has destroyed most Americans' digestive systems. A constant influx of damaged fats and excessive sugars has reduced our collective ability to absorb key nutrients even if we are eating the right kinds of foods. Maximum nutrient absorption is necessary to repair the ongoing damage to the gastrointestinal (GI) tract, or gut.

When looking for a supplement, demand whole food ingredients. Natural ingredients are the most readily absorbed and utilized by the body. The ideal supplement will feature a number of key ingredients, as well as digestive enzymes and a probiotic strong enough to withstand the high acidity levels of the GI tract. Once in the gut, a strong probiotic strain will repair the damage caused by a nutrient-poor diet.[181]

Some of the other featured ingredients should be the essential oils of clove, oregano and thyme. These oils—which should be presented as phenolic compounds—are believed to decrease risk of developing cancers and serve as antioxidants.[182] Clove, oregano, and thyme are all touted for their abilities to ameliorate chronic indigestion, constipation, upset stomach, and other persistent digestive issues. Clove, specifically, soothes inflammation of the intestinal lining by relaxing the smooth muscle fibers, while oregano helps defend against bacterial infections and stimulates white blood cell production.[183, 184] Finally, thyme has long been used to combat intestinal infections due to its strong antimicrobial properties, which deter bacterial, fungal, and viral growth.[185] Combined, the essential oils of these three herbs can restore gut health.

Weight management aid

Even naturally thin people struggle with weight as their hormones shift with age. Added weight increases stress on the systems of your body. An effective weight management aid will support healthy blood sugar levels to keep hormones in check, and will feature natural ingredients to help with stress management. Ideal options will contain no caffeine, and will contain ingredients that help build muscle to improve overall body composition.

KEY CONCEPTS FROM THIS CHAPTER

1. Everyone needs supplementation.

Through some combination of poor diet, nutrient-depleted soil, and genetically modified food, everyone is lacking vital nutrients. These nutrients play critical roles in hormone function, energy production and free-radical protection. Supplementation is necessary to ensure our bodies are equipped with all the nutrients needed to fight disease and function properly.

2. Store-brand supplements offer little or no benefit.

Cheap synthetic ingredients are ignored and quickly expelled by your body, never improving your state of nutrient deficiency. Even worse, these generic vitamins and minerals can accumulate inside your fat cells as toxins. Over time this toxic load builds up, frequently causing new health issues. Conversely, whole-food-based supplements are readily absorbed and utilized by your body.

3. Biomarker testing is essential to overcoming deficiencies.

Everyone has unique nutritional needs. Having a personalized supplementation plan is the smartest method for correcting your nutritional issues. Self-diagnosis can be dangerous, as taking a random assortment of supplements can increase your toxicity. Biomarker testing provides the information needed for a qualified doctor to design the ideal supplementation program for you.

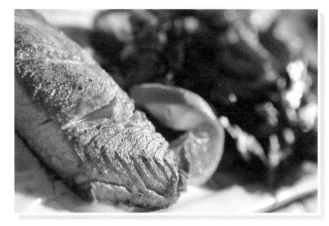

CHAPTER EIGHT:

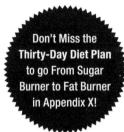

Don't Miss the Thirty-Day Diet Plan to go From Sugar Burner to Fat Burner in Appendix X!

The Maximized Metabolix Diet Plans

A Metabolix food diet that addresses carbs, hormones, inflammation, and aging may sound complicated. But it's not. We've made it so easy a child can follow it. In fact, many do!

In this chapter, you'll find some vital tools, including:

- Your nutrition breakdown on the **Core and Advanced H_2A_2 plans**.

- **Protein counters:** A list of protein-rich foods, how much protein they provide, and how to get 20–30 grams of protein in a single meal.

- **Our carb counter:** A list of foods detailing exactly how many carbs you can expect—with easy-to-measure portion sizes!

- Meal plans that outline exactly what to eat, meal-by-meal, so you can forget about all the "guess work."

- A list of healthy recipes that comply with H_2A_2, allowing you to enjoy desserts and other tasty foods, so you don't feel like you're "dieting."

- Replacement foods—how to change out the wrong for the right.

- Shopping list

- A thirty-day weight loss program to switch you to being a fat burner

Your "New Normal" and the Vacation Rule

The goal of this book is to make your life easier, not harder, to live than it is right now. You'll have to make some conscious decisions to eat better, and that sounds impossible—but I promise you: it's very possible.

When it comes to change, everyone needs it, but no one likes it. That's because any change, no matter how easy it seems, is ultimately tough in the long haul. Eventually, the goal is

The Vacation Rule:

It's not cheating if it's part of the plan!

not to make it hard on yourself, but rather to reach a "new normal."

What's "normal" to you right now is particularly hard to change. But once you've put the right plan in place, it won't be long before it becomes your new normal—a normal that you'll enjoy. Once you're new normal has you looking and feeling so good, you won't want to quit. It's common to resist a new diet because it seems like it means you never get to enjoy life again. So be aware of the "Vacation Rule." This is the "rule" that says that, two or three times each week, you have a favorite food or meal.

None of the recommendations you'll read in this chapter are "Vacation-free." Having one–two "Vacation meals" per week or even an entire "Vacation day" will help make this new change a lifestyle change—and not a death sentence—for your diet.

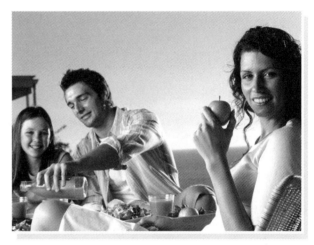

The Vacation idea is simple: having nachos or pizza for lunch once a week, and ice cream on Sunday afternoon, isn't going to hurt. In fact, it

might even help you. And when you go on that Spring Break "Vacation," take a couple of days off the diet. It's mentally healthy—and in some ways, it's even physically healthy.

Because the Metabolix Diet isn't about deprivation—and makes you feel and look so good— you'll be ready to get back to it quickly after "Vacation." What you'll find is that, over time, you choose more and more healthy "Vacation" options because you feel so good with Metabolix foods—and so bad without them.

This is not a typical "die, but with a 't' at the end." Later on, you'll find plenty of recipes for pizzas and desserts—all created with the goal of restoring your hormones to health.

Between tasty, healthy recipes and the Vacation Rule, you're going to create a "new normal" for yourself. Diets don't work if they ask for blood, sweat, and tears. It's when you don't feel like you're sacrificing pleasure that you truly make changes that last.

Advanced and Core H$_2$A$_2$ Plans

Your choices will boil down to one of two plans: the Advanced Plan and the Core Plan. Both follow the three steps in the H$_2$A$_2$ formula.

Advanced

A very low-carb plan. This is for you if you need to lose weight, are potentially insulin resistant/pre-diabetic, or diabetic. The Advanced Plan is also the diet plan for those who are inflamed, in pain, depressed, anxious, toxic, and sick and who require healing. It's the right plan for those with seizures, as well.

This diet radically reduces the troubling inflammation that plagues and ages so many.

One thing we find in our work is that athletes often believe it's the trauma of their sport that causes injuries, when in many, many cases it's actually diet-induced inflammation. They go on the Advanced Plan, and the joints and muscles they thought had damaged become well. As I mentioned previously, I thought my running, wrestling, and competing days were over in my twenties, and I had stopped doing all three. I was a fat-free eating guy, ripped, but I endured continual shoulder, knee, and low back pain. When I traded in my carbs—in the form of oatmeal, pasta, and brown rice—for smoothies, good proteins, berries, vegetables, and avocados, the pain went away completely. As long as I stick with this plan, I can enjoy my hobbies: endurance racing, high-intensity exercise, and mixed martial arts training.

Because carbs are kept low, and you avoid all of the related metabolic shrapnel, people of all ages, health levels, and sizes tend to do very well on the Advanced Plan.

Core

The carbs are still not "high," but they are higher in this plan than in the Advanced Plan so you can do some grains. If you're a healthy individual, with a good carb tolerance, and lead an active lifestyle, follow the Core Plan. If this is your profile, you'll also lose weight or find the optimum weight for you. It's great for kids as, under most circumstances, they can tolerate a higher amount of carbs in their diet.

Following the Plans

Weighing food? Counting calories? Who has time for that? The less math you have to do, the better. In following these plans, there are just two key numbers you will want to pay attention to.

> Approximate grams of carbs per day to fall within the plan using the Carb Counter.

> Approximate grams of protein per meal using the Protein Counter, aiming at 20–30 grams for each meal, three–six times per day depending on your iProtein needs.

Toss out the old "one-size fits all" food pyramids and recommendations, and choose a diet that suits your current status as well as your ultimate goals:

The Advanced Plan

The Advanced Plan is similar to a very low-carb ketogenic diet.

It sounds super-restrictive, but it's not. A cup of strawberries is only 11g of carbs or roughly twenty-five percent of the allotted amount on the Advanced Plan. As described in *Step 1, Curb the Carbs,* you still do get to eat three–four meals a day of carbs depending on portions.

It's not all about deprivation, either. You replace the carbs with fats, proteins, and most importantly, all of the grain-free, properly sweetened, dessert recipes that are so abundant in this plan. Even though it's advanced and causes weight loss, you still get to eat.

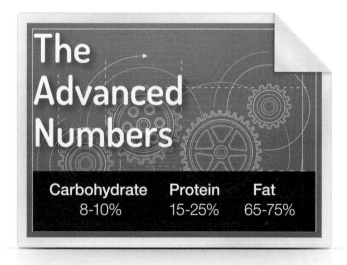

The Advanced Numbers

Carbohydrate	Protein	Fat
8-10%	15-25%	65-75%

On the Advanced Plan, your carb consciousness should be high. Know which number of carbs and which score high on the glycemic index (listed in Appendix III). You can also switch to stevia or xylitol to sweeten foods and use grain-free grain replacements, like flax meal, almond flour, and coconut flour, for baked goods.

Here are some examples of macronutrient breakdowns on the Advanced Plan:

Fast Weight Loss	Active Plan With More Calories	Plan With Poor Access to Quality Protein (Less Protein and Higher Fat)
1,600 total kcal:	2,400 total kcal:	2,400 total kcal:
150g protein (38%)	150g protein (25%)	40g protein (15%)
25g carbs (6%)	50g carbs (8%)	50g carbs (8%)
100g fats (56%)	179g fat (67%)	204g fat (77%)

Once again, your individual plan may vary.

Note: If you don't have access to a lot of protein, it's your fat calories that should go up, not your carb calories.

Stay Encouraged!

As your body becomes more insulin sensitive and tolerant of carbs, you'll be able to move up to the Core Plan, getting 75–100g of carbs a day. On the other hand, many people remain too intolerant of carbs—or just feel too good on this plan—to switch. And again, it's not hard! There are "Vacations"—and the lifestyle can eventually become your "new normal."

The Core Plan

Your macronutrient goals on the Core Plan will break down like this:

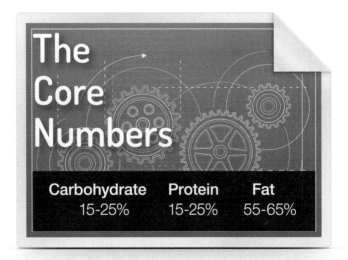

Carbohydrate	Protein	Fat
15-25%	15-25%	55-65%

For Healthy, Active, Carb Tolerant Kids:
25–30% Carbs; 20–25% Protein; and 45–55% Fat

If you aim at taking in around 2000 calories a day, with 15–25% being from carbohydrates, that's 300–500 calories or 75–125 grams. That is a great, carb-conscious lifestyle range.

The 125 grams would be appropriate for a more active individual. The plans we normally recommend contain little to no grains, so Core ends up being closer to 75–100g. This is more along the lines of people's tolerance and allows them to achieve the health and body they so desire.

Definitions

gut noun \'gət\ bomb noun \'bäm\

Calories we put in our body matter, but pale in significance compared to what they do once in our systems. They may not meet our needs most effectively. They may be used, or stored as fat. They may set off a cascade of hormone imbalances, increasing our likelihood of illness and obesity. They may cause inflammation - or prevent it.

Whole, low glycemic foods that are grown or raised properly are readily accepted by the organs of digestion. On the other hand, refined products and foods high in carbs and sugar detonate a gut 'bomb' that blows dangerous metabolic 'shrapnel' everywhere in the system.

A young, active person would likely lose weight and/or get super lean on this plan while an older, more sedentary person will be able to maintain their weight.

Weight loss following this plan is particularly likely if you're only modestly overweight, have put on just a few pounds, and/or are not yet experiencing metabolic symptoms such as high cholesterol or high blood pressure.

Here are some examples of macronutrient breakdowns when you go on a Core Plan diet:

Weight Loss For an Active Individual	2000 Calories	Very Active Individuals
1,800 total kcal:	2,000 total kcal:	2,400 total kcal:
113g protein (25%)	125g protein (25%), 75g	150g protein (25%),
90g carbs (20%)	carbs (15%),	100g carbs (17%),
110g of fats (55%)	133g fat (60%)	155g fat (58%)

Note: These are not hard and fast rules, because each person's macronutrient needs will vary depending on activity level, age, carb tolerance, and body weight. But they are good examples of macronutrient breakdowns that fit within the Core Plan.

Specialized Macronutrient Ranges			
	Carbohydrates	Protein	Fat
An active child	Upper range of carbs: 30%	Upper range of protein: 25%	Lower range of fat 45%
For older adults	Consume the upper range of protein in order to prevent sarcopenia (age-related loss of muscle mass).		
For athletes	Consume the upper range of protein to retain lean muscle mass.		

Don't forget the **Life Risk Questionnaire** at the beginning of the **Appendices**. It will help you to find out which plan and course of action fits you.

"Finally, What I Can and Can't Eat!"

RULE #1.
The Jack LaLanne Rule

Jack LaLanne, a former fitness guru who was still pulling tugboats with his teeth in his 80s, said, "If God didn't make it, I won't eat it."

As I've said, the goal of this book is to make your life easier, not harder than it is right now. The first rule is simply that you eat whole, natural foods, cut way back, or start to eliminate, the grains and sugars in your life, replacing them with better fats and cleaner proteins. Just do that, and you'll see great change. Do the following, and be transformed.

Go Metabolix

Focus on Metabolix Foods. Metabolix foods are whole, low G-I foods.
*(See the detailed Glycemic Index in **Appendix III**)*

Metabolix Foods

- Low GI plant food
- Fruit: Berries, Granny Smith apples, avocados
- Vegetables
- +Omega-3 Foods, including fish, fish oil, flax seeds, flax flour, and chia seeds
- Organic, pasture-raised chicken and eggs
- Grass-fed and finished meat and dairy products
- Olive oil, and coconut oil, flour, and milk
- Key and targeted vitamins and minerals (See **Appendix IV**)

The following foods can be healthy when eaten in moderation. There are metabolic challenges due to certain anti-nutrients that create difficulties with absorption. The grains should be eaten even more sparingly as they are very high glycemic foods.

- **Legumes** (beans, lentils, soybeans, peanuts, and peas), raw nuts, seeds, and nut flour.
- **Small amounts of non-GMO, gluten-free, sprouted grains.** On the Core Plan, some non-GMO grain can be eaten. Supposed non-GMO "ancient grains" are amaranth, quinoa, and millet are gluten-free. Oats are inherently gluten-free, but can be contaminated by wheat during processing. Look for gluten-free oat brands.

Avoid wheat like the plague, including whole or sprouted wheat. Also avoid gluten and gluten-free commercial products—they're generally loaded with processed carbohydrates.
*(See our soaked and sprouted section in **Appendix IX**).*

The Cost:

I know that you might be saying, "These whole foods are expensive; a burger and fries only cost me four bucks. If I want kale, I have to put it on layaway."

However, eating food from a grocery store, particularly the kind of bulk items we mention, is definitely cheaper in the long run than eating out or buying foods that come in a box.

Carbs on the
Core and Advanced Plans

Carbs should be the easiest macronutrient to manage, since you know what your daily goals are. Simply count your carbs and stay within your daily limits, and you've taken care of your carbohydrate business—for the most part.

One word of warning:

No matter which plan you're on, you'll want to switch out high-glycemic carbs for low-glycemic carbs.
*(See the Glycemic Index in **Appendix III**).*

For example, you can switch out red apples for green apples and put almond or peanut butter on celery or green apples instead of crackers.

You can also exchange out wheat flours and start baking recipes that include flax, almond flour, and/or coconut flour. You'll find many recipes in this chapter that call for these flours.

The Carb Counter
A Chart of Lower-Glycemic
Index Carbohydrate Sources

You don't need to abandon carbohydrates to follow the H_2A_2 formula. You just have to know *Step 1—how to Curb the Carbs*. Below, you'll see a list of low-glycemic carbs and how many grams of carbohydrates they have per serving.

It's important to note that, in counting carbs, you can subtract "total fiber" from "total carbohydrates." For example, a cup of blackberries has seven "net carbs" thanks to its 8 grams of fiber.

Because managing your carbs will be integral to your lifestyle whether you're on the Advanced or Core plan, this is an important table:

Food	Serving Size	Total Carbohydrates	Total Fiber
Fruit			
Apples (with skin)	1 medium-sized apple	25	4
Asian Pears	1 whole medium fruit	13	4
Avocado (California)	1 whole, without skin	12	9
Bananas	Medium (7–8" long)	27	3
Blackberries	1 cup	15	8
Blueberries	1 cup	21	4
Dates (Deglet Nour)	1 cup chopped	110	12
Grapefruit	Full fruit (6–8" diameter)	26	4
Grapes	1 cup	16	1
Honeydew melon	1 cup balled	16	1
Kiwis	1 cup	26	5
Lemons	1 fruit	8	2
Limes	1 lime	7	2
Mangoes	1 cup sliced	28	3
Melon (Cantaloupe)	1 cup balled	16	2
Oranges (Florida)	1 large whole fruit	17	4
Peach	1 large whole	17	3
Pineapple	1 cup, chunked	22	2
Plums	1 fruit	8	1

Pomegranate	1 fruit	53	11
Red cherries	1 cup, without pits	19	2
Vegetables			
Artichokes (boiled and prepared)	1 medium artichoke	14	10
Arugula	1 cup, uncooked leaves	1	0
Banana peppers	1 medium whole pepper	2	2
Broccoli	1 cup chopped	6	2
Brussels sprouts	1 cup	8	3
Cabbage	1 cup chopped	5	2
Carrots	1 cup chopped	12	4
Cucumber	1 cup chopped	3	1
Garlic	3 cloves	3	0
Green beans	1 cup	8	4
Green leaf lettuce	1 cup shredded	1	0
Green peas	1 cup	21	7
Jalapeño peppers	1 cup sliced	6	3
Kale	1 cup chopped	7	1
Onions	1 cup chopped	15	3
Potato	1 whole potato	27	2
Pumpkin	1 cup, cubed	8	1
Red peppers	1 medium whole pepper	7	2

Spinach	1 cup, uncooked leaves	1	1
Summer squash	1 cup sliced	4	1
Sweet corn	1 medium ear	26	3
Sweet potato (cooked, with skin)	1 medium whole	24	4
Swiss chard	1 cup	1	1

Nuts and Legumes

Almonds	1 cup whole	30	17
Black beans	1 cup	23	8
Brazil nuts	1 cup whole	16	10
Chickpeas (Garbanzo beans)	1 cup	54	11
Lima beans	1 cup	40	9
Macadamia nuts	1 cup whole	19	11
Peanuts	1 cup	24	12

Low-Glycemic, High-Fiber Grains

Brown rice (cooked)	1 cup	45	4
Multi-grain bread	2 slices	22	4
Oats	1 cup	103	17
Quinoa (cooked)	1 cup	39	5
Rye bread	2 slices	30	4

186, 187, 188

Fat on the
Core and Advanced Plans

If you choose a plan that increases your calories, these additional calories should come from fat rather than carbohydrates. Keeping carbs low and proteins moderate, your main tool for increasing calories will be the fats in your diet.

In the **Advanced Plan**, fats take a major role, making up for low amounts of carbs (as low as 40–100 grams per day, perhaps lower). In the absence of carbs, your body will switch to burning fat, making it a clean-burning source of energy.

In the **Core Plan**, fat also plays a central role in shifting your total caloric intake, though there is more flexibility for low-GI carbs and less reliance on fats for total energy.

Remember Your Oil Change!
Follow Step 2 for the H_2A_2 formula by choosing according to the priority list of fats for your meals.

At 55–77% of the diet, a 2,000-calorie meal plan will have 1,100—1,540 calories of fat. A one-tablespoon serving of oils like olive, coconut, or fish is approximately 120 calories. There are about seventy-two fat calories in a serving of whole milk, forty-five in an egg, and 130 in beef. It won't be hard to go over one thousand calories with a couple of these servings at each of your meals or in your snacks throughout the day.

Protein on the Core
and Advanced Plans

Here are a few reminders for **Step 3** in the H_2A_2 formula—choosing your appropriate iProtein levels.

- Keep your protein at 15–25%.

Calories	15%–25%	Grams
1800	270–450	68–113
2000	300–500	75–125
2400	360–600	90–150
2800	420–700	105–175*

- Lack of organic sources, you are inactive, or chronically ill: 15%
- Clean source and active lifestyle: 25%
- Athletes can move to the "high" side of the equation by adding one or two 20–30g meals or supplemental shakes.

*_**Remember:** this is not intended to be a "high-protein" diet. In a higher calorie diet, unless you're a hard-training athlete, doing a lot of resistance training, and/or a really big dude, 120–150g is a good cap._

Protein Counter

Here's the information you need to help you find how to reach 20–30 grams per meal—as well as hitting your protein goal throughout the day:

Animal foods	
Land	
Beef average	7g per ounce
4 ounces hamburger	28g
6 ounces steak	42g
3 ounces leg of lamb	22g
3 ounces chicken breast, no skin	24g
Sea	
Fish average	6g per ounce
6 ounce can of tuna	40g
4 ounces mahi mahi	20g
4 ounces salmon	24–25g
4 ounces tilapia	23g
3 ounces shrimp	11g
1 ounce sardines	7g
Eggs and dairy	
Large egg	6g
1 cup milk	8g
1/2 cup cottage cheese	15g
1 cup yogurt	8–12g (check label)
Soft cheeses (Mozzarella, Brie, etc.)	6g/ounce
Medium cheeses (Cheddar, Swiss)	7.5g/ounce
Hard cheeses (Parmesan)	10g/ounce
Beans, nuts, legumes, and seeds	
2 tablespoons peanut butter	8g
1/4 cup almonds	8g
1/4 cup peanuts	9g
1/4 cup cashews	5g
1/4 cup sunflower seeds	6g

1/4 cup pumpkin seeds	8g
1/4 cup flax seeds	8g
1/2cup cooked beans	7–10g average

How to Get 20-30 grams of Protein in a Meal

Eggs	4–5 eggs, depending on size
Beef	A 3–4 oz. hamburger patty or beef filet each offers 23–32 grams of protein
Untrimmed steak	3–4 ounces offers 21–28 grams of protein
Leg of lamb	3–4 ounces offers 22–30 grams
Chicken breast, no skin	3–4 ounces offers 24-32 grams
Turkey	3–4 ounces offers 22-30 grams
Mahi Mahi	4–6 ounces offers 20-30 grams
Tilapia	4–6 ounces offers 22.7-31 grams
Salmon	4–6 ounces offers 24-32 grams
Tuna	6 ounce can offers 40 grams of protein
Shrimp	6 ounces offers 22 grams of protein
Milk	Three cups offers 24 grams
Cottage cheese	1/2 cup offers 15 grams
Soft cheeses (Mozzarella, Brie)	6 grams per ounce
Medium Cheese (Cheddar, Swiss)	7–8 grams per ounce
Hard cheese (Parmesan)	10 grams per ounce

How to Read
a Food Label

Law dictates that each food label give you the same information in the same place every single time. That's the good news; it keeps things simple. The bad news is that not all of the information is very relevant, which means you'll have to do a little learning on your own in order to understand which numbers on the food label really matter.

% Daily Value

A child, an adult with diabetes, an endurance athlete, someone who sits at a desk all day, a pregnant mother, and a grandfather all have substantially different nutrient needs. Therefore, the "Daily Values" expressed on food labels are of very little informative value to you. When reading as "% Daily Value" or "%DV," you should ask "Daily Value for whom?"

Total Carbs, Fats, and Proteins

This is good, relevant information, and it's what you need to start checking on all of your food. After listing total calories, the next bolded items include "Total Fat," "Cholesterol," "Sodium," "Total Carbohydrate," and "Proteins."

For the purpose of following the plans, figure out the percentage. Remember, carbs and proteins contain 4 calories/gram and fat contains 9 calories per gram.

Nutrition Facts	
Serving Size 1 cup (228g)	

Amount Per Serving	As Served
Calories 250	**Calories from Fat** 110

	% Daily Value
Total Fat 12g	18%
Saturated Fat 3g	15%
Cholesterol 30mg	10%
Sodium 470mg	20%
Total Carbohydrate 31g	10%
Dietary Fiber 0g	8%
Sugars 5g	
Protein 5g	

Vitamin A 270%	•	**Vitamin C** 10%	
Calcium 2%	•	**Iron** 0%	

Percent Daily Values are based on a 2,000 calorie diet. Your daily values may be higher or lower depending on your calorie needs:

		Calories	2,000	2,500
Total Fat	Less than		65g	80g
Sat Fat	Less than		20g	80g
Cholesterol	Less than		300mg	300mg
Sodium	Less than		2,400mg	2,400mg
Total Carbohydrate			300g	375g
Dietary Fiber			25g	30g

In the image at the right, there are 250 calories made up of:

- Carbs: 31g x 4cal/g = 124 calories
- Protein: 5g x 4cal/g = 20 calories
- Fats: 12g x 9 cal/g = 108 calories

So carbs make up 50% of this food.

Ingredients list

Food manufacturers have to list their ingredients, which means you'll know exactly what you're putting in your body. A good rule of thumb? The fewer ingredients listed here, the better—and if you can't understand the words, don't eat the ingredients.

Serving size

Is another variable to watch out for. You might think a food has few trans-fats, carbs, or calories, only to see that the serving size is the equivalent of a thimble-full.

Looking at the serving size first, located at the top of the food label, helps you understand the overall "context" for all of the numbers printed below.

Manufacturers like to draw your attention away from the nutrition facts by advertising a "healthful" ingredient on the front of the box. They'll tell you all about their product's "whole-grain goodness" or "heart-healthy ingredients." But what they don't advertise are the other ingredients present: processed grains, chemicals, colorings, and enough sweeteners to flavor your swimming pool. Once you read the ingredients list, you have to make a choice:

Beware of Health Claims

A bar tender could claim that a Bloody Mary has lycopene, (a tomato phytochemical) which has been found to lower the incidence of prostate cancer.

However, there are other ingredients in there - such as vodka - that aren't exactly health foods. Cereals made with processed grains, chemicals, colorings, and enough sweetener to flavor a swimming pool will still claim to supply "whole-grain goodness" and be heart healthy.

Too many sugars? Too many carbs? Chemical ingredients? If the answer is yes, just say, "No." Even if the package claims it's healthy.

<h2 style="text-align:center">Your Thirty-Day
Plan for Success</h2>

The following is a thirty-day diet designed to turn you from sugar burner to fat burner, cause you to lose unwanted weight, reduce inflammation, and provide an abundance of health-promoting nutrients.

It begins with three weeks of the Advanced Plan to get you fat-adapted. The meal plans then transition into a more moderately low-carb Core Plan the last week, but without grains. Long term, or if you're very active, you can add grains like brown rice or ancient, gluten-free quinoa to lunch or after exercise.

This process will change your body, your habits, and allow you to get used to living, shopping, cooking, and eating this way. All of the necessary recipes are included with my favorite— plenty of desserts. If you, or someone you know can bake, there's even cheesecake and pizza in the recipe section—just made with Metabolix foods. You definitely can't say you're deprived with this program.

Enjoy the food and the new you.

Meals

You can do exactly as we've placed here or utilize similar, grain and sugar free recipes. If you're OK with leftovers, another great tip is to make enough for multiple meals rather than a new dish virtually every breakfast/lunch/dinner like we've done in the example here.

Snacks and Desserts

Snacks

One way to develop a real carb craving is to get to the point where you're starving and ready to eat a hippo. The key with snacks is to avoid starvation while not adding carbs between meals. The after-dinner snack* should be eaten two–three hours before bed, although vegetables are always free, even right before you sleep.

If your appetite is perfectly satisfied, or you're struggling to lose weight, then you don't need to eat between meals or after dinner, and where the snack options are available, you're not obligated to partake in them.

On the plan we've laid out for you, we provide an example, but below are all of the snack options you can choose from:

Snack Suggestions

- Granny Smith apple, alone or with 1–2 Tbsp almond or peanut butter (Nut butters should have no added ingredients—just the nut.)
- Celery, with 1–2 Tbsp of almond or peanut butter or organic cream cheese
- Vegetable sticks (celery, cucumber, green/red/yellow pepper, romaine) with hummus, Yogurt Veggie Dip,* or guacamole
- Grainless Granola*
- Brownie Cereal*
- 1/2 cup of Greek or goat's milk yogurt, with stevia to taste, shredded coconut, shaved unsweetened chocolate, and ground flax seeds or chia seeds
- Green Smoothie*
- The Dessert Recipes—remember, they're made of nut flowers, good fats, and non-sugar sweeteners, so they're a food.
- Mixed Sweet Nuts*
- Cinnamon Almonds*
- Raw almonds, pistachios, peanuts (on occasion), hazelnuts, and pecans. Cashews are higher glycemic index, suitable for the more active person or the Core Plan
- Salads and leftover cooked proteins and vegetables

The Desserts

Our dessert recipes don't provide many carbs and can be eaten for snacks and after meals. We've placed something sweet after dinner in the plan, but it's not an absolute. Again, if you're satisfied, it's your choice to partake or not. And, of course, while we've named specific dessert examples in the plan, you can choose from the many recipes we've provided.

SUPPLEMENT RECOMMENDATION-
See Chapter Seven for details

- Daily detox supplement
- Vitamin D
- Max GI™—digestive repair
- Daily Defense™—inflammatory support
- Quality omega supplementation

THIRTY-DAY WEIGHT LOSS
Sugar Burner to Fat Burner Plan

	Breakfast	Snack	Lunch	Snack	Dinner
Day 1	Strawberry Smoothie*	Vegetable sticks w/Veggie Yogurt Dip*	Mexican Salad: 6 oz shredded lean cooked turkey with 1/2 cup guacamole, 2 Tbsp organic sour cream, 2 cups chopped tomatoes, and 1 cup chopped onions over 2 cups shredded lettuce	1/4 cup Cinnamon Almonds*	Pepper Steak*, 2 1/2 cups green beans sautéed in 2 Tbsp olive oil and minced garlic, Chocolate Avocado Pudding*
Day 2	Kitchen Sink Yogurt*	3 to 5 sticks celery filled with 1 tbsp. almond butter	Chicken Wings*, 10 celery strips dipped in 1/4 cup sour cream	Green Smoothie*	6 oz salmon grilled in 1 Tbsp olive oil, 2 cups zucchini cooked in 1 Tbsp olive oil, No-Guilt Chocolate Chip Cookies*
Day 3	Chocolate-Covered Strawberries Smoothie*	1/2 cup Cinnamon Almonds*	Green salad with leftover salmon or a 4 oz turkey burger and 1/4 cup olive oil and 3 Tbsp balsamic or white vinegar	No-Guilt Chocolate Chip Cookies*	6 oz grilled chicken, 1 cup chopped cucumber, 1 cup cherry tomatoes, 1 1/2 Tbsp olive oil, 1 tsp balsamic vinegar, Chia Seed Cocoa Almond Pudding*
Day 4	Veggie omelet: 3 eggs, 2 oz organic cheddar cheese, 1 cup mushrooms, 1 cup diced bell pepper cooked in 1 Tbsp raw grass-fed butter, 1 cup blackberries	Medium green apple with 1 Tbsp almond butter	Caprese salad: 4 oz organic buffalo, mozzarella cheese, 2 sliced tomatoes, 2 Tbsp olive oil, 2 Tbsp chopped basil, 1 cup raspberries	Grainless Granola*	Stuffed Bell Pepper*, Salad: Romaine, spinach and/or mixed greens, with any other vegetable, salt, olive oil, basil dressing, No-Guilt Chocolate Chip Cookies*
Day 5	Berry Smoothie*	Vegetable sticks w/Veggie Yogurt Dip*	4 oz Roast Chicken and Cauli-Rice*, 2 cups green beans with 1 Tbsp raw grass-fed butter	Grainless granola*	Chinese chicken salad: 4 oz cooked chicken breast, 2 cups shredded cabbage, 1 1/2 Tbsp sesame oil, 1 tsp rice vinegar 1/2 cup Greek or goat's milk yogurt with stevia, chia seeds, and unsweetened shaved chocolate

*See Recipes in **Appendix X**

	Breakfast	Snack	Lunch	Snack	Dinner
Day 6	Kitchen Sink Yogurt*	Grainless Granola*	Green salad with grilled or baked chicken breast with 1/4 cup olive oil and 3 Tbsp white or balsamic vinegar	Chia Seed Cocoa Almond Pudding*	Warm Steak Salad with Mushroom Brown Butter*, 2 cups chopped cucumber, steamed broccoli, Chocolate Almond Butter Fudge*
Day 7	3-egg omelet with 1 oz organic cheddar cheese, 1 cup mushrooms, 1 cup spinach cooked in 1 Tbsp coconut oil, 2 cups blackberries with 2 Tbsp sour cream	Chocolate Almond Butter Fudge*	6 oz salmon grilled with 1 Tbsp olive oil and garlic, 1 cup broccoli, 1 cup zucchini sautéed in 1 Tbsp raw, grass-fed butter	Green Smoothie*	Protein burger: 4 oz ground grass-fed beef wrapped in lettuce leaves, 1 cup chopped tomatoes with 2 oz mozzarella cheese and 1 Tbsp olive and 1 tsp balsamic vinegar, 1/2 cup Mixed Sweet Nuts*
Day 8	2 Blueberry Muffins*, 1 cup strawberries with 2 Tbsp sour cream	Veggie sticks with guacamole	4 oz lean turkey burger with 1 oz organic Monterey Jack cheese wrapped in lettuce, 1 cup Brussels sprouts roasted with 1 Tbsp olive oil	Chocolate Almond Butter Fudge*	3 oz chicken, 2 cups broccoli, 1 cup cucumbers, 1/2 cup onions sautéed in 2 Tbsp olive oil, 1/2 cup of Mixed Sweet Nuts*
Day 9	3 scrambled eggs cooked in 1 tsp coconut oil, 2 cups spinach cooked in 1 tsp coconut oil and 2 Tbsp water, 1 cup blackberries	Medium green apple with 1 Tbsp almond butter	Chicken Wings*, 1 cup sliced cucumbers and 1 cup cherry tomatoes with 1 Tbsp olive oil and 1 tsp balsamic vinegar	Green Smoothie*	Turkey meatloaf*, Artichoke with 2 Tbsp melted butter, Salad: Romaine, spinach and/or mixed greens, with any other vegetable, salt, olive oil, basil dressing, Chocolate Avocado Pudding*
Day 10	2 blueberry muffins*, 1 1/2 cups blackberries with 2 Tbsp whipped cream and 2 tbsp chopped walnuts	Veggie sticks w/ guacamole	Sardine salad: 4 oz sardines on 2 cups arugula with 2 Tbsp olive oil and 1 tsp balsamic vinegar, 1 oz Brie cheese	Chocolate malted smoothie*	Stuffed Pepper*, Salad: Romaine, spinach and/or mixed greens, with any other vegetable, salt, olive oil, basil dressing, 1/2 cup Greek or goat's milk yogurt with stevia, chia seeds, and unsweetened shaved chocolate

*See Recipes in **Appendix X**

	Breakfast	Snack	Lunch	Snack	Dinner
Day 11	1 cup Greek or goat's milk yogurt with fresh berries and coconut, add xylitol/stevia to taste	Veggie sticks w/ hummus	Chicken Wings*, 2 cups cucumbers, 10 celery strips dipped in 1/4 cup sour cream	Green Smoothie*	5 oz roast beef 1 cup zucchini grilled with 2 tsp olive oil, 2 cups zucchini cooked in 1 Tbsp olive oil, Lemon Squares*
Day 12	Sliced tomato topped with 1/3 cup organic cream cheese and 4 oz salmon, 2 cups raspberries with 2 Tbsp organic sour cream and 2 Tbsp chopped pecans	Medium green apple with 1 Tbsp almond butter	Sardines on romaine lettuce with sliced up hard cheese, tomato, green pepper, and cucumber with 1/4 cup olive oil and 3 Tbsp balsamic or white vinegar	Lemon Squares*	Warm Steak Salad with Mushroom Brown Butter*, 2 cups cucumbers, steamed asparagus, Chia Seed Cocoa Cinnamon Almonds*
Day 13	Strawberry Smoothie*	Brownie Cereal*	Green salad with baked or grilled salmon and 1/4 cup olive oil and 3 tbs balsamic or white vinegar	Sticks of celery filled with almond butter	1/4 chicken, 1 cup chopped cucumber, 1 cup cherry tomatoes, 1 1/2 Tbsp olive oil, 1 tsp balsamic vinegar, faux mashed potatoes, Lemon Squares*
Day 14	Mexican omelet: 3 eggs, 1 cup diced chilies, 2 Tbsp shredded organic cheddar cheese, 2 Tbsp salsa, 1/2 sliced avocado, cooked with 1 Tbsp raw, grass-fed butter, 1/2 cup blackberries	1/2 cup organic whole milk Greek or goat's milk yogurt topped with stevia, ground flax seeds, and shaved dark chocolate	5 oz cold cooked chicken mixed with 1/2 cup guacamole over 2 cups field greens and 1 cup chopped red bell pepper	Green Smoothie*	Green Salad with grilled or baked chicken breast with 1/4 cup olive oil and 3 tablespoons white or balsamic vinegar, steamed broccoli, Cinnamon Almonds*
Day 15	Chocolate Covered Strawberries Strawberries Smoothie*	Vegetable sticks w/ 1/2 cup hummus	Chinese Chicken Salad*	Brownie Cereal*	6 oz chilled tilapia, 3 cups arugula with 2 Tbsp olive oil and 1 tsp balsamic vinegar, chocolate avocado pudding*

*See Recipes in **Appendix X**

	Breakfast	Snack	Lunch	Snack	Dinner
Day 16	1 1/2 cups organic 2% cottage cheese topped with 1/2 cup raspberries and 2 Tbsp chopped pecans	Brownie Cereal*	Sardines mixed with 1/2 cup guacamole over 2 cups baby romaine lettuce, 1/4 cup pecans	4 celery stalks with 2 Tbsp organic cream cheese	Chicken Curry*, salad: romaine, spinach and/or mixed greens, with any other vegetable, salt, olive oil, basil dressing, Coconut Macaroons*
Day 17	2 Grain-free Blueberry Muffins*	Brownie Cereal*	Mexican salad: 6 oz shredded lean ground turkey with 1/2 cup guacamole, 2 Tbsp organic sour cream, 1 cup chopped tomatoes, and 1/2 cup chopped onions over 2 cups shredded lettuce	Green Smoothie*	Stuffed Bell Pepper*, salad: romaine, spinach and/or mixed greens, with any other vegetable, salt, olive oil, basil dressing, Cinnamon Almonds*
Day 18	Chocolate Covered Strawberry Smoothie*	Veggie sticks w/ Veggie Yogurt Dressing*	Green salad with baked or grilled salmon and 1/4 cup olive oil and 3 tbs balsamic or white vinegar	Granny Smith apple with 1 tbsp. almond butter	Grass fed steak broccoli and cauliflower steamed or roasted. Can add Brussels sprouts or other vegetables, Coconut macaroons*
Day 19	2 Grain-free Blueberry Muffins*	Vegetable sticks of your choice with 1/2 cup hummus	Chicken Wings*, 2 cups cucumbers and 10 celery strips dipped in 1/4 cup sour cream	Egg Nog Smoothie*	4oz shredded chicken, 1 cup chopped onion, and 2 cups chopped green peppers cooked in 2 Tbsp, coconut oil, 1/2 cup guacamole, Cinnamon Almonds*
Day 20	Berry Smoothie*	1/2 cup Cinnamon Almonds*	4 oz chicken, 1/2 cup chopped onion, and 1/2 cup green peppers cooked in 2 Tbsp coconut oil, 1/2 cup guacamole	1/2 cup Greek or goat's milk yogurt with 1 oz shaved, unsweetened dark chocolate- Stevia to taste	4 oz chopped grass-fed beef steak, 1 cup broccoli, 1 cup mushrooms, 1 cup chopped yellow bell pepper, stir-fried in 2 1/2 Tbsp coconut oil, Chocolate avocado pudding*

*See Recipes in **Appendix X**

	Breakfast	Snack	Lunch	Snack	Dinner
Day 21	3 scrambled eggs cooked in 1 tsp coconut oil, 2 cups spinach cooked in 1 tsp coconut oil and 2 Tbsp water, 1 cup berries	Veggie sticks w/ hummus	Mexican salad: 6 oz lean ground turkey with 1/2 cup guacamole, 2 Tbsp organic sour cream, 2 cups chopped tomatoes, and 1 cup chopped onions over 2 cups shredded lettuce	1/2 cup Pistachios	Salmon in Basil Cream Sauce*, 1 cup zucchini grilled with 1 Tbsp olive oil, salad: romaine, spinach and/or mixed greens, with any other vegetable, salt, olive oil, basil dressing, Freezer Fudge*
Day 22	1 1/2 cups organic 2% cottage cheese topped with 1/2 cup raspberries and 2 Tbsp chopped pecans	Freezer Fudge*	6 oz cooked chicken breast mixed with 1/2 cup guacamole over 2 cups field greens	Green Smoothie*	Turkey Meatloaf*, Salad: Romaine, spinach and/or mixed greens, with any other vegetable, salt, olive oil, basil dressing, Protein Almond Bar*
Day 23	Chocolate Covered Strawberry Smoothie*	3 to 5 sticks celery filled with almond butter	4 oz chopped chicken breast, 1 cup onions, and 1 1/2 cups green peppers cooked in 1 Tbsp coconut oil, 1/3 cup guacamole	Freezer Fudge*	Salmon or tilapia, mashed faux potatoes, green salad, Avocado Pudding*
Day 24	Kitchen Sink Yogurt*	Protein Almond Bar*	Chinese chicken salad: 4 oz cooked chicken breast, 2 cups shredded cabbage, 1 1/2 Tbsp sesame oil, 1 tsp rice vinegar	Green Smoothie*	Chili: 5 oz ground beef, 1/2 cup tomato sauce, 2 cups diced zucchini, 1/4 cup onions, 1 Tbsp chili powder, 1/2 tsp cayenne pepper, Protein Mixed Sweet Nuts*
Day 25	Strawberry Smoothie*	Vegetable sticks w/hummus	6oz sardines, 3 cups romaine lettuce, sliced hard cheese, 2 Tbsp olive oil, 1 tsp balsamic vinegar	Mixed Sweet Nuts*	4 oz chicken, 1 1/2 cups cherry tomatoes, 1/2 tsp sea salt, and 1/2 cup sliced black olives grilled in 1 Tbsp olive oil, 1/2 cup Greek or goat's milk yogurt with chia seeds, shredded coconut, shaved unsweetened chocolate, and stevia.

*See Recipes

	Breakfast	Snack	Lunch	Snack	Dinner
Day 26	Chocolate Covered Strawberry Smoothie*	Granny Smith apple with 1 tbsp. almond butter	Green salad with grilled or baked chicken breast with 1/4 cup olive oil and 3 Tbsp white or balsamic vinegar	Brownies*	Pepper Steak*, 2 1/2 cups green beans sautéed in 2 Tbsp olive oil and minced garlic, Chocolate Avocado Pudding*
Day 27	Grainless Granola* topped with 1 cup organic whole milk Greek yogurt and 1/2 cup blackberries	3 to 5 sticks celery filled with almond butter	6 oz cooked lean turkey breast mixed with 1/2 cup guacamole over 2 cups baby Romaine lettuce, 1/4 cup pecans	Chocolate Malted Smoothie*	Chicken Curry*, salad: Romaine, spinach and/or mixed greens, with any other vegetable, salt, olive oil, basil dressing, Sweet Mixed Nuts*
Day 28	Berry Smoothie*	1 cup organic whole milk Greek or goat's milk yogurt topped with stevia and 1 oz shaved dark chocolate	4 oz lean turkey burger with 1 oz organic Monterey Jack cheese wrapped in lettuce, 1 cup Brussels sprouts roasted with 1 Tbsp olive oil	1 cup yellow bell pepper strips with 1/3 cup guacamole	6 oz grass-fed ground beef patty wrapped in lettuce leaves, 1 cup zucchini grilled with 2 tsp olive oil, Brownies*
Day 29	Veggie omelet: 3 eggs, 2 oz organic cheddar cheese, 1 cup mushrooms, 1 cup diced bell pepper cooked in 1 Tbsp raw grass-fed butter, 1 cup blackberries	Protein Almond Bars*	Chicken Wings*, 1 cup sliced cucumbers and 1 cup cherry tomatoes with 1 Tbsp olive oil and 1 tsp balsamic vinegar	Green Smoothie*	Chinese Chicken Salad*, Cinnamon Almonds*
Day 30	Chocolate Malted Smoothie*	1/2 cup pistachios	4 oz cold cooked salmon, 2 cups sliced cucumbers, 2 cups cherry tomatoes, 2 1/2 Tbsp olive oil, 1 tsp balsamic vinegar	Granny Smith apple with 1 tbsp. almond butter	5 oz roast beef, 1 cup zucchini grilled with 2 tsp olive oil, Chocolate avocado pudding*

*See Recipes

NOTE: Most days contain 2,000-2,200 calories with a maximum of 2,400. This will put active people at a caloric deficit for the day.

APPENDIX I:

Lifestyle Risk Questionnaire (LRQ)

The LRQ is the ideal way to get an accurate assessment of your current nutritional profile and determine the best place for you to start.

Please check all boxes that honestly apply to you.

1. ☐ Do you exercise less than 3 times a week for 30 minutes at a pace where you are able to carry a conversation with a little strain (i.e. huffing or puffing)?

2. ☐ Are you an athlete that exercises more than 4 times a week for 60 minutes or more?

BODY COMPOSITION

3. ☐ Have you gained 5-10lbs around your midsection in the last six months?
   ☐ Have you gained more than 10lbs in the last year?

4. ☐ Have you had weight gain accompanied by high blood pressure, increased cholesterol and/or uncontrolled blood sugar?

5. ☐ Have you recently attempted to lose weight without success?

YOUR MENU

6. ☐ Do you crave sugar or carbohydrates (ie chocolate, bread)?
   ☐ If so, how often do you experience this craving?
   ☐ Infrequently ☐ Occasional ☐ Daily

7. ☐ Do you crave stimulants (ie coffee or chocolate)?
   ☐ If so, how often do you experience this craving?
   ☐ Infrequently ☐ Occasional ☐ Daily

8. ☐ Are you addicted to caffeine?
   ☐ If so, how often do you consume caffeine?
   ☐ Infrequently ☐ Occasional ☐ Daily

   ☐ Are you addicted to Alcohol?
   ☐ If so, how often do you consume alcohol?
   ☐ Infrequently ☐ Occasional ☐ Daily

   ☐ Are you addicted to Cigarettes?
   ☐ If so, how often do you smoke?
   ☐ Infrequently ☐ Occasional ☐ Daily

9. ☐ Do you eat boxed food more than twice a week?

10. ☐ Do you drink any type of pop/soda?
    ☐ If so, how often do you consume pop/soda?　☐ Infrequently　☐ Occasional　☐ Daily

11. ☐ Do you drink less than 4 glasses of water per day?

12. ☐ Do you eat white flour, white rice or white bread?
    ☐ If so, how often do you consume white flour, white rice or white bread?　☐ Infrequently　☐ Occasional　☐ Daily

13. ☐ Do you eat less than 5 servings of vegetables per day?

14. ☐ Do you use artificial sweeteners like Aspartame, Splenda, and Nutrasweet, or consume foods that contain them?
    ☐ If so, how often do you consume these foods?　☐ Infrequently　☐ Occasional　☐ Daily

15. ☐ Do you eat fried foods more than once per week?
    ☐ If so, how often do you consume fried foods?　☐ Infrequently　☐ Occasional　☐ Daily

16. ☐ Do you eat processed "deli" meat, bacon, sausage, or hot dogs?
    ☐ If so, how often do you consume processed meats?　☐ Infrequently　☐ Occasional　☐ Daily

17. ☐ Do you feel you get all your needed nutrients from food, and therefore pass on supplements including multivitamins and fish oil?

18. ☐ Do you use canola oil, vegetable oil or margarine?
    ☐ If so, how often do you use canola oil, vegetable oil or margarine?　☐ Infrequently　☐ Occasional　☐ Daily

19. ☐ Are most of the fruits and vegetables you eat conventionally grown (non-organic)?

20. ☐ Do you consume milk and dairy products?
    ☐ Do you consume organic/grass fed products?

21. ☐ Are the majority of your animal products from the meat counter or freezer at the grocery store (as opposed to a health food store or local farmer)?

22. ☐ Do you eat sweets or candy?
    ☐ If so, how often do you consume sweets or candy?　☐ Infrequently　☐ Occasional　☐ Daily

23. ☐ Do you drink more than 1 alcoholic beverage, three times per week and/or crave alcohol?

24. ☐ Do you have excessive thirst?

25. ☐ Do you eat wild caught fish less than twice a week?

26. ☐ Do you eat grains (especially gluten) at most meals?

ENERGY

27. ☐ Do you feel your energy and stamina is less than what it has been in the past?

28. ☐ Do you have trouble getting going in the morning, feeling like you need more sleep even if you have gotten 8 hours? ☐ < 8 hours sleep
    ☐ If so, how many hours per night do you sleep on average? ☐ > 8 hours sleep

29. ☐ Do you crave stimulating activities (ie sex, race car driving, sky diving, high velocity biking) to boost your mood and energy? ☐ Infrequently   ☐ Occasional
    ☐ If so, how often do you crave these activities? ☐ Daily

30. ☐ Do you feel like you are running on adrenaline? ☐ Infrequently   ☐ Occasional
    ☐ If so, how often do you feel you are running on adrenaline? ☐ Daily

31. ☐ Do you experience low energy with no motivation? ☐ Infrequently   ☐ Occasional
    ☐ If so, how often do you experience these feeling? ☐ Daily

32. ☐ Do you feel drowsy during the day? ☐ Infrequently   ☐ Occasional
    ☐ If so, how often do you experience feelings of drowsiness during the day? ☐ Daily

33. ☐ Do you have episodes of feeling faint or dizzy or a poor sense of balance? ☐ Infrequently   ☐ Occasional
    ☐ If so, how often do you experience these feelings? ☐ Daily

34. ☐ Do you have anemia (low iron)?

HAIR , SKIN & NAILS

35. ☐ Do you have hair loss, not resulting in baldness (ie noticing more hair on the pillow when you wake, hair loss in shower etc.)?

36. ☐ Do you feel your hair is lack luster?

37. ☐ Do you suffer from eczema and/or psoriasis?
    ☐ If so, which of these conditions do you suffer from?

    ☐ Eczema   ☐ Psoriasis

38. ☐ Do you have acne?

39. ☐ Do you suffer from dry skin and/or dermatitis?
    ☐ If so, which of these conditions do you suffer from?

    ☐ Dry Skin   ☐ Dermatitis

40. ☐ Do your nails have ridges, spots or do they split easily?

SLEEP

41. ☐ Do you have difficulty sleeping, have nervousness or hyperactivity?
    ☐ If so, how often do you experience these symptoms?

    ☐ Infrequently   ☐ Occasional
    ☐ Daily

LIFESTYLE DISEASES

42. ☐ Do you feel you are aging quickly?

43. ☐ Do you have silver amalgams in your mouth?

44. ☐ Do you receive the flu vaccine annually?
    ☐ Have you received the flu vaccine in the past?

45. ☐ Do you live or work in a large metropolitan city that often has smog or heavy air pollution?

46. ☐ Do you have a history of exposure to mold (i.e. living in a home with mold, living in a climate with high incidences of mold, working in older buildings etc)?

47. ☐ Do you have irregular blood sugar, diabetes or pre-diabetes?

48. ☐ Do you have heart disease (ie high blood pressure [over 115/75] or high cholesterol), circulatory problems or slow wound healing?

49. ☐ Do you have metabolic syndrome: obesity, blood pressure over 115/75, diabetes mellitus and high cholesterol?

50. ☐ Do you have a history of cancer?

IMMUNITY

51. ☐ Do you suffer from sinus issues, asthma, or allergies (including rashes, eczema, and hives)?
    ☐ If so, how often do you experience these symptoms?

    ☐ Infrequently   ☐ Occasional
    ☐ Chronic

52. ☐ Do you get frequent colds and flus?

53. ☐ Do you have an autoimmune condition (ie MS, Ulcerative Colitis, Crohn's Disease, Rheumatoid Arthritis, Meniere's Disease, and Raynaud's Phenomenon)?

PAIN

54. ☐ Do you suffer from joint pain or muscle aches?
    ☐ If so, is your pain chronic or infrequent?
    ☐ Infrequently ☐ Occasional
    ☐ Chronic

55. ☐ Do you have headaches or migraines?
    ☐ If so, are your headaches or migraines chronic or infrequent?
    ☐ Infrequently ☐ Occasional
    ☐ Chronic

56. ☐ Have you had a history of whiplash or a concussion?
    ☐ Have you received treatment/correction for your whiplash and/or concussion?

57. ☐ Do you have chronic pain including fibromyalgia or arthritis?

DIGESTION

58. ☐ Do you have any digestive concerns (ie bloating, pain, gas, nausea or excessive body odor)?
    ☐ If so, how often do you experience these symptoms?
    ☐ Infrequently ☐ Occasional
    ☐ Daily

59. ☐ Do you have diarrhea?
    ☐ If so, is your diarrhea chronic or infrequent?
    ☐ Infrequently ☐ Occasional
    ☐ Chronic

60. ☐ Are you constipated? (i.e. less than one bowel movement a day and/or hard difficult stools)
    ☐ If so, is your constipation chronic or infrequent?
    ☐ Infrequently ☐ Occasional
    ☐ Chronic

61. ☐ Do you have alternating diarrhea and constipation?
    ☐ If so, are your symptoms of alternating diarrhea and constipation chronic or infrequent?
    ☐ Infrequently ☐ Occasional
    ☐ Chronic

62. ☐ Do you have hemorrhoids?

63. ☐ Do you have heartburn and/or excessive burping?
    ☐ If so, is your heartburn/excessive burping chronic or infrequent?
    ☐ Infrequently ☐ Occasional
    ☐ Chronic

64. ☐ Do you eat at your desk, while standing or on the go?
    ☐ If so, how often are you eating while standing or on the go?
    ☐ Rarely ☐ Occasional
    ☐ Daily

65. ☐ Have you noticed a recent decrease in appetite?

66. ☐ Do you have skin or nail fungal infections?

MIND

67. ☐ Is your lifestyle what you consider "fast-paced"?

68. ☐ Do you worry, feel stressed, anxious or overwhelmed, especially in typically low stress situations?

69. ☐ Are you irritable?
    ☐ If so, how often do you feel irritable?   ☐ Rarely   ☐ Occasional
                                                    ☐ Daily

70. ☐ Do you feel faint, anxious, irritable or aggressive when you don't eat regularly?

71. ☐ Do you feel sad, depressed, uninterested in daily activities or "down" without an identifiable cause?   ☐ Rarely   ☐ Occasional
    ☐ If so, how often do you experience these   ☐ Daily
       feelings?

72. ☐ Do you like structure and order, even towards the compulsive side?

73. ☐ Do you get seasonal affective disorder (SAD)? (ie low mood in the Winter)

74. ☐ Do you have difficulties with memory, concentraton, lack of focus, ADD, ADHD, brain fog or concerns with behavior?   ☐ Rarely   ☐ Occasional
    ☐ If so, how often do you experience these   ☐ Daily
       symptoms?

75. ☐ Do you lack taking a holiday at least once every 6 months for a week that is relaxing?

76. ☐ Do you work more than 40 hours a week?
    ☐ Do you work more than 45 hours per week?
    ☐ Do you work more than 60 hours per week?

EYES, EARS & MOUTH

77. ☐ Do you have bloodshot, burning or gritty eyes?

78. ☐ Are your eyes sensitive to bright lights?

79. ☐ Do you have loss of hearing?

80. ☐ Do you have a sore tongue?

81. ☐ Do your lips crack easily?

82. ☐ Is your mouth over sensitive to hot or cold?

83. ☐ Do you have bad breath and/or a coated tongue?

LUNGS

84. ☐ Do you experience shortness of breath with mild exertion?

85. ☐ Do you have a history of asthma?
    ☐ If so, how often do you require the use of interventions   ☐ Rarely   ☐ Occasional
                                                                          ☐ Daily
    ☐ (i.e. medication or an inhaler)?

EXTREMETIES

86. ☐ Do you have osteoporosis?

87. ☐ Do you have shooting or tingling in your hands, arms, legs or feet?
    ☐ If so, how often do you experience these symptoms?   ☐ Infrequently   ☐ Occasional
                                                            ☐ Chronic

88. ☐ Do you have a hot or burning sensation in your feet or tender heels?
    ☐ If so, how often do you experience these symptoms?   ☐ Infrequently   ☐ Occasional
                                                            ☐ Chronic

89. ☐ Do you have muscle cramps, tremors or spasms?   ☐ Infrequently   ☐ Occasional
    ☐ If so, how often do you experience these   ☐ Chronic
      symptoms?

90. ☐ Do you have muscle weakness (unrelated to strenuous exercise)?
    ☐ If so, how often do you experience these symptoms?   ☐ Infrequently   ☐ Occasional
                                                            ☐ Chronic

91. ☐ Do you have weak ligaments and tendons? (ie bursitis, tendonitis, frequent injuries to the joints)   ☐ Infrequently   ☐ Occasional
    ☐ If so, how often do you experience these   ☐ Chronic
      symptoms?

92. ☐ Do you have restless leg syndrome?

93. ☐ Do you retain water or feel "swollen"?
    ☐ If so, how often do you experience these symptoms?   ☐ Infrequently   ☐ Occasional
                                                            ☐ Chronic

FEMALE

94. ☐ Do you take hormonal contraceptives (ie the birth control pill, patch, hormonal creams or Norplant)?
    ☐ If so, have you previously used hormonal contraceptives?

95. ☐ Do you take synthetic estrogen medication? (ie Estratab, Menest, Premarin, Premphase and Prempro)

96. ☐ Have you had difficulties in conceiving or experienced miscarriages?

97. ☐ Do you have Pre-menstrual Syndrome (PMS)? (ie breast tenderness or water retention, mood changes, discomfort or pain)?

98. ☐ Do you or have you had fibrocystic breasts, uterine fibroids, or cervical dysplasia?

99. ☐ Do you have vaginal infections, urinary tract infections, rectal itching or vaginal itching?   ☐ Infrequently   ☐ Occasional
    ☐ If so, how often do you experience these symptoms? ☐ Chronic

100. ☐ Are you peri-menopausal or menopausal? (ie changeable periods, hot flashes, heavier periods, changeable moods)

MALE

101. ☐ Do you feel like you have lost your competitive edge?

102. ☐ Do you feel reduced sexual performance or libido?   ☐ Infrequently   ☐ Occasional
     ☐ If so, how often do you experience these symptoms? ☐ Chronic

103. ☐ Do you or have you had prostatitis or benign prostatic hypertrophy?

104. ☐ Do you have a history prostate cancer?

105. ☐ Do you have difficulties with urination?
     ☐ If so, how often do you experience these symptoms?   ☐ Infrequently   ☐ Occasional ☐ Chronic

106. ☐ Have you had difficulties with fertility?

107. ☐ Do you snore or have sleep apnea (stop breathing at times or gasp during the night)?   ☐ Infrequently   ☐ Occasional
     ☐ If so, how often do you experience these symptoms? ☐ Chronic

WHAT'S YOUR SCORE?

Your Doctor will review your answers and assign a score based on the information you provided. Your score indicates your level of risk and will help determine where you need the most support.

SCORING:

60+: Crisis/Highest Risk

Health crisis that requires immediate implementation of the Advanced Plan, metabolic testing and targeted therapeutic nutrients to recover from metabolic damage that has already occurred.

51-59: Pre Crisis/High Risk

Areas present that require immediate attention; lifestyle and eating habits have been contributing to ongoing metabolic dysfunction which has the potential to create serious health consequences. It's important to address this dysfunction immediately with the Advanced Plan, metabolic testing and targeted nutrients.

41-50: Moderate to High Risk

Areas present that require immediate attention as they have the potential to develop into worsening conditions. Address specific conditions, lifestyle, nutritional shortcomings and nutritional deficiencies. A more aggressive approach is required like the Advanced Plan, metabolic testing and targeted nutrients to achieve a lower score within 6 months.

31-40: Moderate Risk

Improvements needed to address the early, potential development of nutritional deficiencies

11-30: Moderate to Low Risk

Minor improvements to diet and lifestyle, ensuring basic nutrients are being met through supplementation and Core Plan Principles

10 or less: Low Risk, but Lifestyle Modifications will still result in improvement

SUMMARY

You are better off moving in the right direction slowly than the wrong direction quickly. As you may have guessed all of the items on the list are problematic when it comes to being healthy. Sadly, North Americans hold the dubious honor of having the unhealthiest diet on the planet, as well as the most lifestyle-related diseases, such as heart disease, diabetes, high blood pressure and cancer. So if you've found problems, you're not alone. You're also not without hope. We've helped thousands just like you change their health, transform their body, and experience Maximized Metabolix.

Your Initial Nutrition Review
in Our Office Includes:

- Personalized Dietary Assessment to determine which nutritional plan is right for you.
- Overview of the Maximized Living Nutrition Plans
- Fundamental supplementation guidelines and recommendations, if necessary
- Review of our local Shopping Guide

APPENDIX II:

The "Fat is Bad and Carbs are Good" Myth

To break out of the "fat is bad and carbs are good" mode of thinking, think along the lines of Maximized Metabolix. Ask these kinds of questions:

- What will the calories in your body do?
- Will they meet your nutritional needs?
- Will they be utilized as fuel or stored as fat?
- Will they upset your body's hormonal balance?
- Will they require the production of insulin to keep blood sugar stable, an effect that may one day lead to your cells growing less sensitive to the hormone?
- Will they be accepted by your organs as good fuel or detonate a "gut bomb" that leaves metabolic shrapnel everywhere?

The Failure of Low-Fat and Reduced-Calorie Diets to Create Real Weight Loss

Below is just a sample of the available research comparing low-carbohydrate to low-fat diets. While there is certainly a bunch of literature out there supporting benefits to a lower fat diet, answer honestly: if lowering your dietary intake of fat were the answer to weight loss, wouldn't we be thinner and healthier by now? After all, "low fat" has been the traditional nutrition and medical recommendation for four to five decades.

Low-Fat and low-carb: Which Diet Really Works Better?

In 2003, a study in the New England Journal of Medicine found that restricting calories and fat was less effective for weight loss in obese subjects than was simply restricting carbohydrates.[189]

In 2004, a study had 120 volunteers split up: one group would try a very low-carbohydrate diet (known as the ketogenic diet) without calorie restriction, while the other would stick to a low-fat, low-calorie, low-cholesterol diet. The study, published in Annals of Internal Medicine, concluded that "compared with a low-fat diet, a low-carbohydrate diet program had better participant retention and greater weight loss." Additionally, the low-carb dieters saw their cholesterol panels improve more than did the low-fat, low-cholesterol group.[190]

A **2008** study comparing the low-carb, higher fat Mediterranean diet with the low-fat diet found that the low-fat diet was least effective in producing weight loss. Meanwhile, the low-carb diet had the "more favorable effect on lipids."[191]

A **2009** study found that their low-carb dieters reduced their Body Mass Index more significantly than the low-fat dieters.[192]

Another Question to Consider

If low fat eating was the proper plan, then why do low-carb, higher fat diets work so well? If the conventional wisdom was correct, these studies should have turned out very differently.

If "eating fat makes you fat," then the subjects on the low-carbohydrate diet should not only have lost less weight than their fat-and-calorie-restricted counterparts, but they should have gained weight.

Something is making us fat—but it's not the fat in our diets.

The physiological bottom line to any physical issue, including weight gain and obesity, is that you have to address root biological causes and not just treat symptoms. Cutting the fat and calories doesn't get to the underlying causes of why the body gains weight and why you can't keep it off.

The "Fat = Disease" Myth

If the fat in our diet isn't making us fat, maybe it's not making us sick, either. One thing we know for sure: fat is not the metabolic villain we once thought it was.

Long-term studies with large sample sizes have also shown that low-fat diets did little to nothing to improve the health of their subjects. One study of post-menopausal women, calling itself the "largest long-term, randomized trial of a dietary intervention ever conducted to our knowledge," found that a low-fat diet only led to an overall weight loss of 0.4 kilograms compared to a control group.[193] What's more, the study found that there was no appreciable difference in risk of stroke, cardiovascular disease[194], invasive breast cancer[195], or colorectal cancer.

All of this science, of course, wasn't available when the US Dietary Guidelines were first published in the late 1970s. In 1977, a Senate committee recommended that Americans lower their fat intake—especially animal fat intake—and replace the calories with carbohydrates. These guidelines were not released with total agreement within the scientific community, however.[196] Instead, they were published with a significant degree of controversy, including some researchers claiming that more study was needed before any recommendations could be made to the American public.

It looks like those who wanted more studies done were correct. The 1977 Dietary Guidelines have influenced a generation of parents, teachers, and doctors, helping contribute to much of the same "conventional wisdom" that is making it so difficult to find positive results from low-fat diets in this day and age. We've gotten used to how bad things have gotten with our health and just continue to accept the current nutrition paradigm as good dogma.

Go to any grocery store and you'll see that conventional wisdom still reflected in the packaging and marketing of low-fat or low cholesterol products, many of which are packed full of sugar, starch, and chemicals. Americans listened to the dietary guidelines, flocked to the stores, and bought "health" food that was actually bad for them. Who can succeed at losing weight when they're not getting the right information?

Maybe we haven't been failing at our diets. Maybe our diets have been failing us.

How Did We Get Here?
A Brief History of
Bad Diet Advice

Fat wasn't always considered a dietary devil. For a long time, it was more or less common knowledge that foods rich in carbohydrates were the true culprits driving obesity.

In fact, you can go back and read Jean Anthelme Brillat-Severin's nineteenth-century work *The Physiology of Taste* (which also includes the famous aphorism, "Tell me what you eat, and I will tell you what you are," which later became "You are what you eat"). In the book, he reached the conclusion that restricting starches and sugars would help reduce body fat. *Dr. Spock's Baby and Child Care* offered the same conclusion as early as the 1940s.[197, 198]

Then, in the latter twentieth century, something changed. Much of the shift in conventional wisdom may have been due to the work of a researcher named Ancel Keys, particularly a research project known as the "Seven Countries Study." The study reviewed heart disease information and compared it with the average calories from fat in each country's diet. The results appeared to show a strong correlation between fat in the diet and rates of heart disease. Keys' conclusions received so much attention that he even appeared on the cover of Time Magazine.[199]

If fat was indeed more dangerous than once thought, then eaters across the world would have to get their calories elsewhere—most specifically, through carbohydrates. Less than two decades after the Seven Countries Study appeared, the US government officially recommended that Americans get most of their calories from carbohydrates, while limiting their dietary fat and cholesterol intake.

There was just one problem. Ancel Keys' work—and much of the dietary research of the twentieth century—was controversial. Many of Keys' contemporaries reacted skeptically to his conclusions, including Jacob Yerushalmy, a Berkley statistician, and Herman Hilleboe, the

New York Commissioner of Health.[200] They published a strong criticism of Keys' conclusions, even using Keys' own data to demonstrate associations between higher fat intake and lower mortality rates. (Of course, these were only associations, as well, and didn't prove that fat is healthy any more than Keys had proved that fat was unhealthy).

Even so, it wasn't long before the fat-as-culprit theme took off. The same thing happened for cholesterol in the diet, even though Ancel Keys himself believed that dietary cholesterol had an insignificant impact on blood cholesterol.

The full story of how we arrived at today's dietary myths can fill a book on its own. But suffice it to say, the media reported the shaky science, the culture listened, and consumers clamored for low-fat options in their grocery stores.

Beef was out, and baking was in.

Calorie "Mythbusters"

In 2006, a review was published in the American Journal of Clinical Nutrition that examined the results of eighty-seven weight loss studies. Their conclusion? "Low-carbohydrate, protein above normal low, baseline recommendations diets favorably affect body mass and composition independent of energy intake."[201]

That phrase—independent of energy intake—is very powerful. It means that study subjects lost weight not as a result of how many calories they took in. If "a calorie is a calorie is a calorie," weight loss should occur no matter what types of calories are consumed. But that's not what the science shows us.

Advancements in nutrition science have made it abundantly clear that the macronutrients you eat have varying effects on your body. Different foods affect hormones, cells, and genes in different ways. This, in turn, affects how the body absorbs, moves, and stores the food. It's not really about taking in less energy or expending more—rather it's about the metabolic impact of the food you take in, or what we call "Metabolix."

The types of fuel you ingest enter into different metabolic pathways in order to be broken down safely. There's a "downstream" reaction for each different type of nutrient, with varying degrees of effects on our health. Some promote health and leanness while others cause inflammation, form triglycerides, damage hormone receptors, and cause you to get out of shape.

Even intuitively, we understand that one hundred calories from an apple will affect our body differently than one hundred calories from a candy apple. One will have a higher glycemic index, raising our blood sugar higher and requiring more insulin to control. If you're diabetic, you're all too aware of this effect.

The notion that "a calorie is not a calorie" was recently tested by researchers at Boston Children's Hospital, led by Dr. David Ludwig.[202] The researchers fed their subjects diets with the same amount of calories—only some diets were higher in carbohydrates and some in fats.

As it turned out, the people who ate a diet lower in carbohydrates ended up effortlessly expending more calories than those on a low-fat diet. Subjects on the low-fat diet needed to exercise for an hour a day to match the calories expended by those on the low-carbohydrate diet.

If you're overweight, it is important to simply lose weight. Yet the truth is, not all weight-loss is created equal. It's better to lose pounds from fat than pounds from muscle. You can be thin and unhealthy. Your body composition matters. In fact, your muscle-to-fat ratio is one of the most important measurements of your health.

Having more muscle on your body is healthier for a number of reasons. More muscles helps in glucose uptake, which helps your body manage its blood sugar. One study found that muscle mass is inversely correlated with insulin resistance.[203] Added muscle can also raise our basal metabolic rate.

Consider the long-term study of post-menopausal women quoted earlier, by the Women's Health Initiative. Over seven years, the average weight lost on a low-fat diet was only one pound. And yet the average waist circumference—one way to measure belly fat—increased. This suggests that the subjects didn't only fail to lose body fat, but may have gained more fat than they lost muscle.[195]

Answer honestly: if you could embark on one of two diets, one that burned more fat and one that burned more muscle, which would you choose? Most sane people would choose the fat-burning diet, the one that improves body composition without compromising lean muscle tissue. That should be the goal of any plan.

APPENDIX III:

Carbohydrates and Insulin:
The Dirty Secret of Nutrition

Insulin Action

For insulin to work, it binds to a receptor at the surface of the muscle cells. This allows the glucose in your blood to be transported across the cell membrane and into the cell to be used for energy or to replace depleted glycogen levels in the muscles and liver.

In the case of most people, they're simply not active enough to utilize the glucose stored in the liver and muscles. So their glucose tank is on "full." All of that sugar you digest is processed slowly.

At the same time insulin is promoting glucose movement into the muscles, it's inhibiting glucose production and output from the liver. All of this is done in a vital effort to keep blood sugar levels stable.

Insulin also affects the fat cells. It has to do something with the excess glucose, after all—it can't make it simply vanish. So insulin turns to stored body fat. In fat cells, it shuts off the fat release button and promotes the intake of fatty acids, fat storage, and triglyceride synthesis. So, in the case of insulin resistance, insulin fails to perform these critical functions. Instead, without the glucose transport system being turned on by insulin, the glucose is left to hang out outside the cell, ultimately causing hyperglycemia.

Nothing good can happen from there: there will be conversion of glucose to fat, increased inflammation, and higher cholesterol. The rise in insulin then causes more fat to be locked up (because, after all, that's what insulin does) and a meteoric increase in excess stored fat baggage.

Imagine if you're insulin resistant—what happens if you continue to eat 200–300+ grams of carbohydrates a day? You'll get more hyperglycemia, more fat production, more fat locked into cells, more fat stored, more triglyceride formation, more inflammation, and more disease.[204]

In this book, you learned that carbohydrates are the chief dietary stimulant of insulin, a growth hormone required for the cells to process sugar and that promotes fat storage and prevents fat burning.

We all have a different tolerance to the carbohydrates in our diet based largely on our individualized insulin response. This becomes crucial to the food choices you need to make. Insulin creates fat and also locks it in storage rather than allowing it to be burned for energy. As you lower carbs, and therefore insulin, the benefits are clear—and proven.

Addressing Insulin Resistance
Finding Your Carb Tolerance

Insulin resistance is a condition that worsens or improves over time, depending on whether you're continuing to pile on the carbs and releasing insulin, or cutting back the carbs. This means the carbohydrates you can tolerate now are not necessarily the same amount of carbohydrates you could tolerate as a child—or even a year or two ago.

At one extreme, you have 300g/day. Unless you're super-active or extremely carb-tolerant, you're likely on your way to a problem. On the other hand, you have the Very Low-carbohydrate Ketogenic diet which can cause you to lose weight and can help type 2 diabetics reduce their dependence on drugs and insulin .

When you find your "carb zone," you should notice that you lose weight and feel better as the inflammation and oxidation diminishes. If applicable, you'll see other symptoms of Metabolic Syndrome, like high blood pressure or low HDLs, improving.

Carbohydrate tolerance is highly individualized. Many people can lose weight eating a moderately low-carb diet of 300–500 carb calories or 75–125 grams of carbohydrates per day. Others may need the more serious intervention of a very low-carbohydrate diet, also known as a ketogenic diet of under 200 carb calories, or less than 50 grams a day. To put it into perspective, a Starbucks Frappuccino has 65g of carbs all by itself!

The current "My Plate" Recommended Daily Amounts of carbohydrates includes about 45–65% of your total calories, or potentially well over 300 grams of carbohydrates per day. That's a whole lot of insulin!

There is a different carb-tolerance level for everyone. If you've gotten too far along the path of insulin resistance, just about any level of carbohydrate in your diet can be hazardous to your health. Other people can seemingly deal with all of the cookies and pizza they want—at least for now.

The Physiology of
Becoming a Fat Burner
Going Ketotic

What happens when you stop eating so much glucose? If you eat few enough carbohydrates, your body will make the shift to ketosis, which means:

The brain uses glucose from glycogen stored in the liver. Glycogen in the muscles is used by the muscles.

Your body makes up additional energy requirements through gluconeogenesis. It makes sugar out of protein and a little out of fat. This isn't a great long-term solution as eventually the protein it will utilize could be from the muscles and organs themselves. Thankfully, the body's natural survival mechanism switches to raising ketones for energy instead.

Your body shifts to producing ketones. By synthesizing substances from fatty acids (and to a lesser degree amino acids) to produce ketones, your body now has an alternative energy source that, after a few weeks, can supply a major portion of energy to the brain and the nervous system.

The goal is to shift your primary source of fuel to fat rather than glucose. This happens when you switch to 50g of carbohydrates or less/day in response to the reduction in insulin. While we raise protein above the standard survival RDAs, this is not a high protein diet as excessive protein can convert to sugar.

At this level of carbohydrate intake, after two to three weeks, the primary ketone (beta-hydroxybutyrate, or B-OHB) will rise above a near non-existent baseline present in someone eating the generally recommended 300 grams or more of carbs a day. The keto-adapted, fat burner's liver will now produce ketones at a level of 1–3 millmolar (mM).

Above 1mM, the preponderance of the brain's energy now comes from ketones. The remaining energy will come from the glucose you do take in from your 50g of carbs or less and through gluconeogenesis in the liver.

You don't have to stay here forever. While many people find they do very well with, or can only tolerate, this type of carb limit, which still includes three to four servings of different carbs per day depending on portions, once you adapt to burning fat, you can move to a 75–100g/day range.

Low-carb Diets and Health:
The Science

Randomized Controlled Trials Studying Low-carb Diets Compared with Other Diets

Study results	Where Published?
A systematic review of clinical trials studying low-carbohydrate diets found that low-carb diets were associated with the following: • Decreases in body weight • Less inches around the waist • Improved blood pressure (both systolic and diastolic) • Improved triglycerides • Improved fasting blood glucose • Increased HDL • No significant change in LDL • "Favourable effects on body weight and major cardiovascular risk factors"	Obesity Review, 2012[205]

Subjects on the low carblow-carbohydrate diet lost the most weight (nine pounds on average) and saw the most **favorable** effects on blood lipids, compared to the Mediterranean diet and a low-fat diet.	The New England Journal of Medicine, 2008[206]
The very low-carbohydrate lost both more weight and body fat, and had normal levels of blood pressure, lipids, and insulin.	The Journal of Clinical Endocrinology & Metabolism, 2003[207]
"Severely" obese subjects lost more weight and saw more favorable effects on insulin sensitivity and triglyceride levels even **after** adjusting for the amount of weight lost. They lost more weight than subjects on a low-fat diet.	The New England Journal of Medicine, 2003[208]
Both low-fat and low carblow-carb subjects lost weight, but the low carblow-carb subjects lost more.	The Journal of Pediatrics, 2010[209]
The low carblow-carb subjects lost more weight and had improvements even in non-HDL cholesterol levels. Study was conducted on overweight adolescents.	The Journal of Pediatrics, 2003[210]
The low carblow-carb, ketogenic diet subjects improved hemoglobin, bodyweight, and HDL cholesterol.	Nutrition & Metabolism, 2008[211]
The very-low-carbohydrate, high-saturated fat diet had beneficial effects on "most of the CVD risk factors measured," just as the other diet did.	The American Journal of Clinical Nutrition, 2008[212]
Compared with a low-fat diet, low carblow-carb subjects had better triglycerides and HDL cholesterol.	The American Journal of Clinical Nutrition, 2009[213]
The high-fat, low-carb subjects saw better weight loss, weight circumference, and triglycerides.	The Journal of Clinical Endrocrinology & Metabolism, 2005[214]
Premenopausal, overweight, and obese women eating low carblow-carb lost more weight and "experienced more favorable overall metabolic effects" than those on the Zone, Ornish, or LEARN diets.	Journal of the American Medical Association, 2007[215]

As the science is beginning to show us, you don't have to have a low-carbohydrate tolerance to see the health benefits of a low-carbohydrate, high-fat diet. A 2006 study[216] found that diets lower in carbohydrates improved your cholesterol profile, even when you were not losing weight and, yes, still eating saturated fat.

On the other hand, the review also noted that low-fat diets required the presence of weight loss in order for their health benefits to occur.

Insulin in Fat Storage

In addition to managing blood sugar levels, insulin is involved in several key metabolic processes. Insulin is also known as the "fat hormone" as it plays many roles in the regulation of fat tissue:

Insulin's Role	Effects
Increasing esterification of fatty acids	Boosts your body's ability to turn fatty acids (not body fat) into triglycerides (body fat)
Facilitating lipogenesis	Helps your body create triglycerides for use in body fat
Inhibitor of HSL and ATGL	Prevents burning of body fat for fuel

As you'll notice, none of these roles of insulin are anything you're normally looking for when it comes to body composition.

In small amounts, rises in blood sugar don't do much damage. But when your system is overwhelmed with sugar from carbohydrates, your body stores the energy as fat. In the process, a number of other unhealthy metabolic events occur.

High Fructose Corn Syrup

High fructose corn syrup isn't quite the same as sugar—it may be worse. Products sweetened with high fructose corn syrup will certainly contribute to an overproduction of fat and issues with digestion and digestive organs—like contributing to fatty liver disease.[217]

So while lower on the glycemic index, substantial or regular fructose consumption is associated with an increase in obesity.[218] Consistent fructose intake may also cause insulin resistance,[188, 219] as some research suggests. There is evidence that sucrose and high-GI food intake may also increase the risk of colorectal cancers.[220] Some other research suggests that increased fructose may lead to small intestine and esophageal cancers in older people.[221]

A hormone specialist at the University of California-San Francisco School of Medicine named Dr. Robert Lustig has taken a particular interest in high-fructose corn syrup, arguing that the chronic intake of fructose through sugar and HFCS so prevalent in the diet are not only primarily to blame for obesity and diabetes rates, but may actually be chronic toxins."[222]

Foods to Avoid:

Want less fructose in your diet? It's as simple as reading the ingredients list and avoiding foods that contain sugar (glucose and fructose) and high fructose corn syrup. But don't be surprised to see high fructose corn syrup everywhere, from soda pop to bread.

Lustig even went so far as to say that a high-sugar diet is, in fact, a "high-fat diet" because of the action of fructose in helping generate fat.

This all goes to show that not all sugars are alike, and perhaps the very worst type of sugar (one high in fructose) is becoming a common ingredient in everything from sweetened soda to the bread we eat.

What's more, studies published in both Environmental Health and the Institute for Agriculture and Trade Policy assert that levels of mercury were detected in high fructose corn syrup in many common, name-brand foods. Realize that there is no safe level of mercury to ingest.

More on Fiber

Fiber is generally touted as healthy for two good reasons. First, fiber increases stool size and can help prevent constipation. Second, additional fiber in the stomach can slow the rate at which your stomach is emptied, which in turn slows the metabolic effects, like the insulin response, of the food you're eating.

Fiber is part of most all plant, whole foods. As a result, there are many other good side-effects, like an association with lower cholesterol and reduced risk of colon cancer.

You can find fiber in fruits, vegetables, nuts, seeds, beans, legumes, and whole grains. (Preferably, you'll want these soaked/sprouted—see our Appendix IX for how to do this.) There are two types of dietary fibers: those that dissolve in water and those that don't. Each type of fiber can offer unique health benefits.

Insoluble Fiber, or "Roughage"	Without dissolving in water, your body puts this fiber with the rest of your stool, making it larger and preventing constipation. This has the side effect of speeding up the rate of digestion, or "moving your bowels." You might consider insoluble fiber to be nature's laxative.
Soluble Fiber	The fiber that does dissolve in water plays the part of slowing down digestion, particularly in delaying the emptying of food from your stomach to the small intestine. This can lead to better blood-sugar management, as sugar that stays in the stomach longer is not absorbed as quickly into the bloodstream.

The Glycemic Index

Glycemic Index of Foods:
High Fiber Vegetables:
The "Free Foods"

Food	Glycemic index (glucose = 100)	Serving size (g)
Vegetable (per 100 grams cooked)		
Brussels sprouts	16	100
Cabbage	10	100
Cauliflower	15	100
Celery	15	100
Green Beans	14	100
Lettuce (average)	10	100
Mushroom	10	100
Onion	10	100
– 100+		
Green peas, average	51	80
Carrots, average	35	80
Parsnips	52	80
Baked russet potato, average	111	150
Boiled white potato, average	82	150
Instant mashed potato, average	87	150
Yam, average	54	150
Sweet corn, boiled	60	80
Beetroot	64	80
Pumpkin	75	150
Beans, Legumes		
Broad beans	79	80
Baked beans, average	40	150
Black-eyed peas, average	33	150
Black beans	30	150
Chickpeas, average	10	150
Chickpeas, canned in brine	38	150
Navy beans, average	31	150
Kidney beans, average	29	150
Lentils, average	29	150
Soy beans, average	15	150
Cashews, salted	27	50
Peanuts, average	7	50

Food	Glycemic index (glucose = 100)	Serving size (g)
Grains & Pulses		
Pearled barley, average	28	150
Couscous, average	65	150
Quinoa	53	150
White rice, average	89	150
Quick-cooking white basmati rice	67	150
Brown rice, average	50	150
Converted, white rice (Uncle Ben's®)	38	150
Whole wheat kernels, average	30	50
Bulgur, average	48	150
Lentils (green), average	32	150
Lentils (red), average	26	150
Rye, average	34	150
Millet, average	71	150
Processed Cereals		
All-Bran™, average	55	30
Coco Pops™, average	77	30
Cornflakes™, average	93	30
Cream of Wheat™ (Nabisco)	66	250
Cream of Wheat™, Instant (Nabisco)	74	250
Grapenuts™, average	75	30
Muesli, average	66	30
Oatmeal, average	55	250
Instant oatmeal, average	83	250
Puffed wheat, average	80	30
Raisin Bran™ (Kellogg's)	61	30
Special K™ (Kellogg's)	69	30
Breads		
Bagel, white, frozen	72	70
Baguette, white, plain	95	30
Coarse barley bread, 75–80% kernels, average	34	30
Hamburger bun	61	30
Kaiser roll	73	30
Pumpernickel bread	56	30
50% cracked wheat kernel bread	58	30
White wheat flour bread	71	30
Whole wheat bread, average	71	30
100% Whole Grain™ bread (Natural Ovens)	51	30
Pita bread, white	68	30

| Corn tortilla | 52 | 50 |
| Wheat tortilla | 30 | 50 |

Food	Glycemic index (glucose = 100)	Serving size (g)
Noodles & Pastas		
Fettuccini, average	32	180
Macaroni, average	47	180
Macaroni and Cheese (Kraft)	64	180
Spaghetti, white, boiled, average	46	180
Spaghetti, white, boiled 20 min, average	58	180
Spaghetti, whole meal, boiled, average	42	180
Corn pasta	78	180
Instant noodles, average	47	180
Durum wheat noodles, average	52	180
Mung bean noodles	33	180
Rice noodles, average	53	180
Dairy Products & Alternatives		
Milk, full fat	41	250ml
Milk, skim	32	250 ml
Soymilk, full fat, average	40	250ml
Soymilk, reduced fat, average	44	250ml
Yogurt, average	36	200g
Reduced-fat yogurt with fruit, average	33	200g
Soy yogurt	50	200g
Custard, home-made	43	250ml
Ice cream, regular	57	50g
Ice cream, premium	38	50g

Food	Glycemic index (glucose = 100)	Serving size (g)
Processed Snacks & Beverages		
Coca Cola®, average	63	250 mL
Fanta®, orange soft drink	68	250 mL
Gatorade	78	250 mL
Corn chips, plain, salted, average	42	50g
Fruit Roll-Ups®	99	30g
M & M's®, peanut	33	30g
Microwave popcorn, plain, average	55	20g
Potato chips, average	51	50g
Pretzels, oven-baked	83	30g
Snickers Bar®	51	60g
Chicken nuggets, frozen, reheated in microwave oven 5 min	46	100g
Pizza, plain baked dough, served with Parmesan cheese and tomato sauce	80	100g
Pizza, Super Supreme (Pizza Hut®)	36	100g
Cakes & Pastries		
Banana cake, made with sugar	47	60
Banana cake, made without sugar	55	60
Sponge cake, plain	46	63
Vanilla cake made from packet mix with vanilla frosting (Betty Crocker®)	42	111
Chocolate cake made from packet mix with chocolate frosting (Betty Crocker®)	38	111
Pound cake (Sara Lee®)	54	100
Croissant	67	60
Donut (cake type)	76	60
Blueberry muffin	60	60
Apple muffin, made with sugar	44	60
Apple muffin, made without sugar	48	60
Waffles, Aunt Jemima (Quaker Oats®)	76	35
Banana cake, made with sugar	47	60
Shortbread	64	25

Source: health.harvard.edu

WHY IS FRUCTOSE LOW GI?

Fructose is a type of sugar similar in chemical structure to glucose, but with a much different physiological impact. Fructose produces a smaller rise in blood glucose and serum insulin after eating than other common carbohydrates, i.e., it has a lower GI than foods that only contain glucose. However, there is the concern that fructose increases blood levels of lipids.[223] Fructose is taken directly to the liver where it is immediately metabolized; some is converted to sugar, but most fat. Therefore, small doses of fructose, such as those found in fresh fruits, are considerably more beneficial. The fructose levels in fruits don't raise blood sugar substantially, and the small amount blended with fiber won't create any significant fat production or issues with digestion.

APPENDIX IV:

Weight Loss and
Weight Loss Resistance (WLR)

Here are the other areas of Weight Loss and Weight Loss Resistance to help you get fit or get past challenges to getting lean and dropping weight.

- Testosterone
- Stress and sleep (which affect hormones)
- Cortisol
- Intensity and duration of exercise
- Toxins

Testosterone

If you've ever heard commercials on the radio promising you testosterone treatments that will make you strong, young, and energetic, then you know the appeal of increasing testosterone. The best way to get more of it is to increase production in your own body.

Testosterone

Testosterone is an anabolic (building, or growing) hormone. It builds muscle and burns fat.

Some of the Roles of Testosterone Include:
Maintaining a healthy distribution of body fat.
Increasing muscle strength, thereby preserving lean tissue during weight loss.
Helping produce red blood cells, which may help the body to heal injuries.
Source in the body: Sex organs.

Health Comments

- Low testosterone is correlated with a number of ill health effects, the most notable of which can include low sex drive and belly fat.
- Low testosterone can also raise estrogen.

Here are some ways you can bring testosterone back up:

 Work out first thing in the morning, before breakfast.

 Do shorter, high-intensity workouts like Max T3—which you'll learn about soon. Long-duration, low-intensity exercise can raise bad hormones and lower the good ones.

 Eat low-carb. Men eating a low-fat diet saw decreased testosterone when compared to their usual, higher-fat diets, according to a 2005 study.[224] What's more, a 2013 study found that ingesting pure glucose lowered testosterone in the blood almost immediately.[225] It's no wonder that a diet lower in fat seemed to reduce testosterone levels in men.

Resistance-based exercise. Moving heavy objects will help you increase testosterone. According to a study published in 2010,[226] an acute testosterone response has a big role in explaining why resistance training helps muscle hypertrophy, or muscle growth. You can find out more about exercise in Appendix VII.

Get your vitamin D3. Did you know vitamin D can affect testosterone levels? A 2011 study found that men taking vitamin D saw a "significant increase" in testosterone levels over a group merely taking a placebo.[227]

Intense exercise. See the section on "Max T3" in the fitness appendix to learn all about how to tackle intense exercise without overdoing it on our next hormone, cortisol.

Cortisol

Cortisol is getting more and more attention lately, and with good reason. As a "catabolic" hormone, cortisol could be considered testosterone's "evil twin." Rather than building muscle and burning fat, it breaks down tissue and promotes fat. When cortisol is high, you become a fat-building, muscle-burning machine.

Cortisol's role is to aid us in the "fight-or-flight" response—those tense situations of stress when we need readily-available energy. In the process of being ready to punch or run, cortisol suppresses other systems, like immunity, in order to give us the strength we need to deal with an enemy.

As a hormone, cortisol is here to help us—but it doesn't do that when it's misused. Being in fight mode while sitting at your car, computer, or tossing and turning in bed is a hormonally bad fitness choice.

Cortisol

Cortisol is considered by many to be the "stress hormone." In modern society, we encounter more stress—and more cortisol—than we were meant to handle.

Cortisol Plays a Role in Our Metabolism and:
Increases "gluconeogenesis," or glucose-creation, in the body's systems, increasing available, ready-to-burn energy
Chronically-high levels of cortisol can lead to the loss of lean muscle tissue[228]
It suppresses immunity.
Source in the body: The adrenal cortex. Unsurprisingly, cortisol is often released to deal with acute stress, just as adrenaline is.

Health Comments

- Given that cortisol causes an increase in blood sugar, chronically high levels can be associated with insulin resistance–it's no wonder stress causes us to gain weight!
- A 2010 study demonstrated that low-calorie dieting increases cortisol.[229]

Cortisol management requires going beyond the diet:

Exercise. In addition to exercise's physical benefits, it has the added benefit of reducing chronic stress. Shorter duration, higher intensity exercise causes less overall stress to the body and helps with other hormones like testosterone and insulin sensitivity as well.

Mental relaxation. A 2009 study researched the relationship between guided imagery aimed at reducing stress and cortisol levels in adolescents and found there was indeed a correlation.[230]

Sleep! The average person is getting over 300 hours less sleep per year than is necessary to avoid the stressful effects of deprivation.

Hug! Good relationships reduce stress levels and reduce cortisol.[231]

Toxins

A "toxic load" can spoil your attempts to lose weight (as well as cause inflammation and oxidation).

Toxins ...

- Slow your metabolic rate.
- Disrupt pH in the stomach, blood, and tissues.
- Disrupt absorption of minerals.
- Disrupt hormonal activity due to changes in receptor sites.
- Lower thyroid function.
- Bind to fats making them tough to lose.

Whole Food

The more you focus on eating whole, physiologically-sound foods, the less you'll have to worry about additives.

While most food additives and similarly-related toxins won't have a noticeably acute effect, it's the chronic effects you need to worry about. Overall, you'll want to limit your exposure to the following:

Medications	By design, they change bodily function. They're the purest definition of toxin and as a result, always have side-effects. Get healthy, and with the help of your doctor, reduce or get off the drugs.
Plastics	Avoid plastic containers and water bottles with BPA. All plastics contain dangerous phthalates you'll want to avoid. Store and heat food and drink using glass or stainless steel containers.
Polystyrene	Styrofoam cups, plates, and food holders contain this chemical, which gets into foods, especially when they've been heat.

Tap water	Chlorine, bacteria, heavy metals, and other toxins are found in unfiltered sink and shower water.
Artificial sweeteners	You thought sugar was bad, but artificial sugars are worse. Aspartame and sucralose are two of the most common sweeteners to avoid.
Personal care products	From aluminum in your deodorant to chemicals in your sunscreen, be aware of what you put on your body on a daily basis.
Fluoride	Added to the water supply and tooth products for stronger teeth, fluoride has also been associated with cell membrane damage and potential hormone issues.
Heavy metals	You wouldn't eat lead, mercury, cadmium, or arsenic, but it's possible to find these in exhaust, medications, amalgam fillings, and personal hygiene products.
Food additives	Everything from dyes and colors to preservatives.
DEA or diethanolamine	Found in beauty products and shampoos, DEA has been found to inhibit brain function in mice in high enough amounts.[232]

** If you want to find out more about how to minimize toxins in your environment, check out **Appendix VIII**, which includes a section on food additives and toxins to avoid. Also look at the supplement **Chapter Seven** on the best way to find good detox support.*

STRESS AND SLEEP

Getting Enough High-Quality Sleep

Many people struggle with lack of sleep. The National Sleep Foundation says a majority of American adults don't get eight hours of sleep on a nightly basis, with the daily averages only approaching eight hours on the weekends.

This wouldn't be bad news if we didn't know that lack of sleep can have negative consequences on the hormone concentrations in your body.

Eve Van Cauter, a sleep researcher at the University of Chicago, once conducted a

How to Get Better Sleep

Eve Van Cauter, a professor at the University of Chicago, recommends you find out your own sleep needs by sleeping as much as you can the first few days of your next vacation.

With your "sleep debt" cleared, you can then see how much your body naturally sleeps over the next few days.

Find an approximate average, and you then know how much sleep you need every night.

study to see how sleep (and lack thereof) changed the hormone levels in young, healthy men. After just two nights of less sleep, she found that sleep-deprived men had 18% lower leptin and 28% higher ghrelin levels in their systems. One subject reported being so hungry that he would have "eaten my pillow." It's no wonder—lack of sleep appears to create a hormonal recipe for increased appetite.

That's why it's not surprising that another study, conducted by Stanford University and the University of Wisconsin, found similar hormonal results (increased ghrelin, lower leptin) amongst those who got less sleep—not to mention a higher BMI for those who regularly slept less than 7.7 hours.

There's only one conclusion: if you want to lose weight, sleeping well is one of the most important things you can do. If you're eating well, but not losing weight, turn off the reality TV shows and go to bed.

Exercise Intensity

Your health is multi-faceted. Therefore, to improve health, attention must be paid to nutritional habits as well as several other factors. This is why physicians commonly recommend healthy diet and exercise as an unofficial prescription for hundreds of general health problems.

Where high quality food can increase energy levels, balance blood sugar, and reduce the amount of toxins entering your body, exercise bolsters each of these benefits—and many more.

Physical fitness boosts the body's ability to take in and utilize oxygen, just as whole-foods nutrition boosts the body's ability to absorb and utilize nutrients. Exercise in general helps maximize the body's ability to function and helps improve body composition (a ratio of muscle-to-fat).

While traditional cardiovascular exercise, like jogging on a treadmill or cycling does burn calories, the length of time required to complete such a workout can actually have negative effects. This long-duration exercise can actually cause the body to begin storing calories as fat, as it triggers the production of the stress hormone cortisol. Once the body realizes the workout will not be over soon, it makes cortisol to store energy for future long-distance jogs or bike rides.

On the contrary, short-duration exercise that requires brief bursts of near-maximum effort does not initiate the release of cortisol. Instead, this high-intensity interval training boosts resting metabolic rate via the "afterburner effect," also known as excess post-exercise oxygen consumption (EPOC). This effect encourages the body to continue burning calories for up to two full days after a workout has been completed. Combined with high quality nutritional habits, intense short-duration exercise can drastically improve body composition. As body composition improves, lean muscle increases. As a result, the body can also detoxify more effectively.

Additional Weight Loss Resistance and Health Recovery Resistance Tips

Here are a few additional nutrition tips for WLR that you should know. Good news: they are also incorporated into our diet plans.

Restoring a Normal Metabolism

Tip	Why Does it Work?
Restrict or avoid wheat-, barley-, and rye-based products. In addition to the insulin response these foods will create in your system, there's evidence that they'll actually change the way your body responds to leptin.	WGA, or wheat germ agglutinin, will bind with leptin receptors—which, of course, prevents **leptin** from binding to these receptors and doing what it's supposed to do, which is regulate your body fat and appetite. The science of this effect is still young, but at least one study has shown WGA to inhibit leptin binding.[233]
Avoid fructose. As if you needed another reason to avoid fructose, there is an emerging hypothesis that fructose's role in leptin resistance is another major reason it's causing so many of us to become metabolically out of whack.	A 2011 study in the British Journal of Nutrition compared a "Western-type diet" to a high-fat diet in rats. Unsurprisingly, the high-fat diet was not shown to increase leptin resistance, but the diet high in fructose *did*.[234] The correlation was so close as to "suggest that fructose is the bioactive of a [high-fat]/high-sugar diet that is essential for the induction of leptin resistance." That's a powerful statement for the role of sugar in obesity.
Watch your triglycerides. No, not the fat in your diet, but the triglycerides in your blood. Because high triglycerides are a biomarker for a range of other health problems, you should be doing this anyway—but there's also evidence these triglycerides affect more than just the heart.	Why keep blood triglycerides low? It's simple: they "decreased the transport of leptin across the BBB," or "blood-brain barrier," according to a 2004 study in *Diabetes*.[235] This means that the leptin produced by your body fat in order to keep your body lean is physically prevented by triglycerides in the blood. High-fat, low carblow-carb diets, you'll recall, are particularly good at lowering blood triglycerides, thereby maximizing the effect of the leptin in your blood. That may be one reason low carblow-carb diets allow you to eat as much as you want: they also serve as natural appetite regulators.

APPENDIX V:

Vitamins and Minerals

Meet the *micronutrients*. Vitamins and minerals are not rich in energy like carbohydrates and fats are, but they are rich in essential nutrients that your body cannot live without. The micronutrients in your diet might be small, but they're vital.

Vitamins

As you saw in the previous sections, the definition of an "essential" nutrient kicks in not only when your body needs a nutrient for its own health, but when your body is also incapable of synthesizing the nutrient on its own. Thus far, the essential nutrients you've met are two fatty acids and nine amino acids.

Some people look at vitamins as something you and your kids may or may not need from your "One-a-Day" or "Flintstones Chewables." Yet vitamins are essential compounds. If you go below minimal levels, disease and even death are possible. As with all essentials, the optimum levels are critical for health and longevity, so these should be taken seriously.

There are two types of vitamins: those that dissolve in fat and those that dissolve in water.

The Fat-Soluble Vitamins

The vitamins that dissolve in fat and the vitamins that dissolve in water have very different destinies in your body. Most specifically, the fat-soluble vitamins can be stored, while water-soluble vitamins are easily excreted from the body via urination.

Fat-soluble Vitamins:
Vitamins A, D, E, K,

Fat-soluble vitamins can remain in the body longer. While it's possible to over-consume them, most people are radically deficient in these important micronutrients.

The Water-Soluble Vitamins

Looking at the list of water-soluble vitamins leads to an obvious question: why are there so many B-vitamins? Originally, B vitamins like thiamin (B1) and folic acid (B9) were considered all part of the same

Water-soluble Vitamins:
Vitamins C and all B-vitamins

vitamin—"Vitamin B." But as the science progressed, the research showed that they are each distinctive enough to be viewed as separate vitamins.

Because water-soluble vitamins can leave the body so easily via urine, it's important to make sure that you're getting enough.

Minerals

As is the case with vitamins, essential minerals vary widely in what they do for your body and how much you actually need of each.

- **Essential Minerals.** There are seven essential minerals that your body needs in order to maintain health. You're likely familiar with a few of them, like potassium and sodium. But other essential minerals—like magnesium and phosphorus—are still important.

A Major Role

Micronutrients like vitamins and minerals might only be necessary in small quantities, but they play a major role in your health and diet.

- **Trace Minerals** like zinc and iron aren't needed in such high quantities, but they're still crucial for a range of bodily functions.

There's more to the story of the small substances that appear in your food, because not all "micro" food is friendly. In this section, we'll not only explore the small nutrients that can help keep you healthy, but the small toxins that appear in far too many modern grocery products—and how to avoid them.

Vitamins Explained

The earliest medical miracles were vitamins. Scurvy, rickets, pellagra, beriberi, birth defects, osteoporosis, and many other conditions were "miraculously" cured when we simply figured out that these illnesses were associated with specific vitamin deficiencies. No other medical breakthrough has come even close the important discovery of micronutrients.

Today, while there is still some resistance within the medical community, many scientists, doctors, and athletes have learned to rely on vitamins, minerals, and other nutrients as causes and solutions to health problems.

If lack of a key nutrient can cause a serious disease—or even kill you— then an inadequate supply of key nutrients will clearly impede health and performance. As much, even though the complete absence of a vitamin will become evident with the diagnosis of a disease, deficiencies can arise over time without notice and lead to illness. These illnesses will be treated with drugs, or may even confuse doctors, but could be prevented or alleviated through the right amount of nutrients.

The Fat-Soluble Vitamins

Vitamin	Potential Health Benefits	Deficiency-caused Diseases and Problems
A	Bone growth, reproduction, cell functions, vision, immune system[236]	Night blindness, anemia
D	Calcium absorption, bone health, osteoperosis prevention[237], immunity, mood (hormones)	Osteomalacia, or rickets; increased risk of osteoporosis, auto-immune
E	Antioxidant, immunity, gene expression[238]	Myopathy, Dysarthria, retinopathy, immune system damage

| K | Necessary for blood clotting, bone health in the elderly[239] | Poor blood clotting, bleeding, heavy menstruation, increased risk of cystic fibrosis |

The Water-Soluble Vitamins

Vitamin	Potential Health Benefits	Deficiency-caused Diseases and Problems
Bp	Sometimes simply referred to as "choline," but essential for bone growth, reproduction, cell functions, immune system, hair growth	Liver disease, atherosclerosis, and possible neurological disorders
B1	Cell membrane health, neurotransmission	Beriberi and optic neuropathy
B2	Digestion, immune system, vision	Cracked lips, sore throat, anemia
B3	Red cell production, body growth[240], brain health	Metabolic slow-down, pellagra
B5	Improving cholesterol, joints[241]	Apathy, fatigue, and irritability
B6	Skin health, treating arthritis, wound healing[242]	Anemia, nerve and skin damage
B7	Cognitive function, cardiovascular health	Conjunctivitis, numbness and tingling and the extremities
B9	Hair/fingernails, diabetes prevention, skin rashes in infants[243]	Neural tube defects in utero, which can lead to spina bifida
B12	Cancer prevention, reduced cardiovascular disease risk, reduced stroke risk[244]	Mania and psychosis in severe cases, increased risk of dementia
C	Nerve health, blood cell health, anemia prevention, collagen health[245]	Scurvy, general ill health

Whole Food Sources of Vitamins

While nature has provided us with plenty of whole foods that offer vitamins in abundance, many things have led to modern nutrient deficiencies. Food processing, nutrient-robbing foods, toxins, indoor/sedentary lifestyles, modern agriculture, and diets that have become grain-based, rather than plant-based, have all contributed to a culture of vitamin- and mineral- deficient people.

Like a sailor avoiding scurvy, it's important for you to make sure you have all of the micronutrients you need. Between whole "phoods" and a targeted supplement program specific to your needs, you can be fully nutrient-ized and avoid the all-too-common symptoms and conditions of nutrient deficiencies.

Here are some good sources of fat-soluble vitamins A, D, E, and K:

Vitamin	Whole Food and Natural Sources
A	Carrots, spinach, red peppers, cantaloupe, broccoli, beef liver
D	Exposure to sunlight, fish liver oils, fatty fish, milk, egg yolks
E	Sunflower seeds, almonds, hazelnuts, peanuts, spinach
K	Spinach, collard greens, broccoli, Brussels sprouts, cabbage

Fat-Soluble Vitamin Supplementation Guide:
A, D, E, & K are stored both in the liver and in your body's fat. These are stored longer, so should be more difficult to develop diseases caused by vitamin deficiencies. It also means vitamin toxicity can be an issue as they aren't so easily passed from the body. However, because of today's poor diet and the other factors we listed that create deficiency, fat-soluble vitamins are generally lacking in the bodies of modern men, women, and children.[246] These common fat-soluble deficiencies have a pronounced impact on today's modern, chronic illnesses. One study showed that supplementation of vitamin E caused a 34% reduction in heart attacks and a 49% reduction in cardiovascular death.[247]

In the case of vitamin D, there are a whole host of medical problems that may related to low vitamin D levels, from heart disease and autoimmune disease to cancer. While traditional medical paradigms are beginning to realize the importance of vitamin D, they often recommend a level as low as 400IU per day. We recommend more, sometimes as high as 4000–5000IU per day. A paper published in Pharmacotherapy in 2012 found that "the decision by young, otherwise healthy adults to take vitamin D in doses of 2000 IU/day or lower is unlikely to cause harm."[248]

Heart disease, autoimmune disease, cancer, and many seemingly unrelated illnesses have been linked to vitamin D levels.[249, 250]

It's vitally important to test your levels of vitamin D in your blood. Usually, the "normal" rating is 30ng/ml per day, but many sources point to a minimum of 50ng/ml. We've had success with our patients aiming for 60–80 ng/ml (100–150nmol/L).
(For those with sarcoidosis, hypercalcemia is possible at even normal doses and vitamin D serum ranges).

Here are common food sources for **water-soluble vitamins:**

Vitamin	Whole Food and Natural Sources
Bp (Choline)	Milk, animal liver, eggs, peanuts
B1	Beef and pork liver, milk, eggs kale, cauliflower, potatoes
B2	Milk/dairy, green leafy vegetables, eggs, almonds, cheese
B3	Protein sources including meat, fish, and poultry, and offal
B5	Chicken, beef, tomatoes
B6	Beef liver, tuna, salmon, chickpeas
B7	Offal (organ meats, especially liver), egg yolk, Swiss chard
B9	Leafy green vegetables, avocados, milk, beets, turnips
B12	Meat including poultry and fish, yogurt, milk
C	Oranges, strawberries, broccoli, red and green peppers

251, 252, 253

Water-Soluble Vitamin Supplementation Guide:

Water-soluble vitamins can only be stored in small amounts, which is why the overload will pass out of your body. This is why it's possible to become deficient in water-soluble vitamins in just a short amount of time if you aren't continually reinforcing your body's supplies.

Other issues, like stress, also cause B-vitamin depletion, so a B-complex or multi-vitamin is a pretty standard need. Because B12 is found primarily in animal products, however, vegetarians often have issues getting enough. Since your body easily disposes of excess amounts of water soluble vitamins, over-supplementation is generally not a concern.

A Note on RDA and RDI Numbers

You may notice a distinct lack of RDA and RDI numbers in this section. Why? The Recommended Daily Allowance (RDA) and Recommended Daily Intake (RDI) numbers you see on a regular basis are largely misunderstood. They're very old guidelines created as minimum recommendations to avoid nutritional diseases like scurvy and rickets. Unfortunately, they don't give you a lot of information about what constitutes a healthy amount of micronutrients for you.

Although the RDAs have been revised occasionally, they still essentially act as minimum recommendations. They also don't tell you anything about what you need during pregnancy, with illnesses, for times of stress, athletics, or a whole host of variables that separate your nutritional needs from the nutritional needs of your neighbors.

Consider the case of vitamin E. The RDA for vitamin E is only about 15mg/day, or about 22IU. Yet one study found that an amount of 100–200mg/day helped endurance athletes.[254] Another study found those who took 400IU of vitamin E daily showed a 41% reduction in heart disease, a 22% reduction in death from cancer, and a 27% decrease in all-cause mortality.[255] It's unlikely that you'll get these ideal levels of vitamin E without supplements.

If those numbers seem a little "out of whack" to you, then you know why RDAs and RDIs aren't always effective measurements of the vitamins and minerals you need in your diet.

Minerals Explained

As you learned earlier in this appendix, there are two types of minerals in your diet: essential and trace minerals. Really, all of these nutrients are essential for health and vitality—the difference being that the "trace" minerals are required in much smaller amounts. Let's start by taking a look at the essential minerals.

Essential Minerals

Mineral	Role in Health	Common Food Sources
Potassium	Along with sodium, potassium regulates ATP, a critical element of metabolism	Bananas, avocados, sweet potatoes, yogurt, yellow-fin tuna
Chloride	Hydrochloric acid production in the stomach	Table salt, seaweed, tomatoes, celery, olives, lettuce
Sodium	Regulates ATP along with potassium	Table salt
Calcium	Critical for tissue health, including muscle, heart, bone, and digestive system	Spinach, dairy: milk, yogurt, hard cheeses
Phosphorus	Bone health, cellular health, energy processing	Dairy, meat, eggs, peas
Magnesium	Bone health, heart function, ATP processing, and a strong role inflammation and obesity[256], relaxant, energy production Magnesium deficiency is an extremely common and dangerous condition.	Brazil nuts, pumpkin seeds, almonds, halibut, green leafy vegetables

As for those chemical elements you need in small amounts—but still need—let's have a look at what are called trace minerals:

Trace Minerals

Mineral	Role in Health	Common Food Sources
Zinc	Essential for several metabolic enzymes	Red meat, seafood
Iron	Essential for protein and enzymes including hemoglobin	Eggs, beef, lentils

Manganese	Enzyme and energy functions	Nuts, beans/legumes, teas
Copper	Enzyme function	Nuts, seeds, seafood
Iodine	Essential for hormone production	Iodized salt, some seaweed
Selenium	Enzyme function, including antioxidant enzymes	Brazil nuts, organ meats, seafood
Molybdenum	Function in enzymes regulating nitrogen, carbon, and sulfur cycles	Legumes, nuts, eggs, sunflower seeds

It's worth noting that another element, fluorine, is considered by many to be an essential trace mineral in the form of fluoride, thanks to its teeth-strengthening benefits.

Common Causes of Vitamin and Mineral Deficiencies

Given the importance of these micronutrients, it's not surprising that the less you get, the more likely you are to get sick. Here are some of the most common causes of vitamin and mineral deficiencies:

- **Phytates:** Prevalent in plants and seeds, phytates can reduce the absorption of calcium, magnesium, and iron. They bind to these minerals and make them insoluble, which is another way of saying "indigestible." Additionally, the zinc in whole grains is poorly absorbed into the blood because it's bound tightly to phytates.
- **Oxalic acid:** Common in spinach and can bind to calcium, leading to poor absorption. Kale and broccoli have higher absorption rates for their calcium, making them a superior source. Spinach has value, so don't avoid it altogether—but limit to a few days a week.
- **Medication:** Medications are not without their side effects. B12, magnesium, folic acid, and calcium deficiencies are common and dangerous effects of medications. One example is the statin drugs. Statin drugs can lower your zinc, which in turn creates a wide range of problems because over two hundred zinc-dependent enzymes are affected. Zinc, in general, is critical to cell function and immunity. Statins can also deplete your selenium, which is a valuable mineral. Its deficiency can lead to prostate or thyroid problems, cancer, and an inability to detoxify the daily load of chemicals that hasten disease and aging. Additionally, it's been discovered that the vitamin-like substance CoQ10, which plays an important role in energy production and cardiovascular function, can be depleted by these meds.
- Other common examples are **birth control pills** which deplete B6, B12, and folic acid and diuretics which deplete valuable heart minerals like magnesium.
- **Sweat:** Everything from exercise to illness can cause problems with absorption and deficiency. Sweating will also increase your need for electrolytes, or essential elements.

Naturally Micronutrient-Rich Foods to Eat Regularly

Eating foods that offer a variety of these essential vitamins in every serving is always the starting point to maximizing micronutrients.

Here are some of "nature's multivitamins":

Avocados	Rich in vitamins K, C, B5, B6, dietary fiber, monounsaturated fat, and even potassium, avocados are one of the first places to look for low-glycemic nutrition.
Eggs	Particularly the yolks. Vitamin B2, B5, D, B12, Bp, iodine, selenium, protein—eggs just about have it all, which is one reason why they're such a popular breakfast food.
Nuts	Nuts like almonds, hazelnuts, Brazil nuts, and walnuts perform particularly well when it comes to minerals. In fact, Brazil nuts are so rich in selenium that it's recommended you don't overdo it and enjoy just a few at a time. You'll recall from earlier on that nuts can also provide essential fats.
Green Leafy Vegetables	Whether it's kale, spinach, mustard greens, Swiss chard, or collard greens, it's hard to go wrong adding a serving of green leafy vegetables to a meal. Green leafy vegetables are rich especially in vitamin K, but they also contain lots of Vitamin A, manganese, magnesium, iron, and vitamin C.
Salmon and Other Fatty Fish	One of the rare foods very rich in vitamin D, salmon is no slouch when it comes to other vitamins like B3 and B12. Fatty fish in general are fantastic sources of nutrition.
Broccoli	Just about any green vegetable could appear on this list, but broccoli is such an important food that it deserves a section all its own, offering vitamins C, K, and A as well as a number of B vitamins in smaller amounts. Just a cup's worth of broccoli has more than one hundred percent of your daily value of vitamin C.

Phytochemicals:
Reduce Cancer Risk,
Inhibit Inflammation,
and More

Vitamins and minerals aren't the only nutritional assistance offered by natural foods. One area of research that shows a lot of promise is that of phytochemical study.

"Phytochemicals" refer to substances contained in plants like fruits and vegetables that may be able to help prevent diseases and illness.

The basic theory is simple: plants utilize a large number of chemicals that help protect them from the wild—from too much sun, from pests, from weather, etc. In some cases, these basic protections extend to us when we consume the plants' phytochemicals.

How is this possible? Much of it has to do with the hormonal action of these nutrients, as well as the stimulation of specific enzymes in our body.

Indoles, the phytochemicals found in cabbages, stimulate enzymes reduce the risks associated with estrogen, thus potentially reducing the risk of breast cancer.

Allicin, found in garlic, has anti-bacterial properties.

Some phytochemicals will bind physically to cell wells, making it harder for pathogens to adhere to them. **Proanthocyanidins** in cranberries, for example, perform this task, which may be why they help fight urinary tract infections and improve dental health.

There are so many phytochemicals in nature, however, that it's impossible to catalog them on a table as you might with vitamins and minerals; the table would take up an entire college-length text. Some estimates say there are over 40,000 phytonutrients that will eventually be cataloged. By enjoying a diet rich in fresh vegetables, fruits, and green tea you are exposing yourself to 5000–10,000 phytonutrients every day!

Eat Plants

The impact of many of these nutrients has been found to fight free radicals, reduce the risk for certain cancers, and improve important functions like immunity and managing inflammation. Here are some of the most important phytochemicals known to science thus far:

Phytochemical	Source(s)	Biological Function in Humans
Beta carotene	Carrots	Powerful antioxidant
Lycopene	Tomatoes	Powerful antioxidant, improves immune function
Lutein and zeaxanthin	Spinach	Improves immunity and helps fight cancers
Anthocyanins	Blueberries and grapes	Antioxidant, anti-inflammatory
Quercetin	Apples, citrus fruit, onions	Antioxidant, anti-inflammatory
Indoles, glucoinolates, and sufloraphane	Cruciferous vegetables (broccoli, Brussels sprouts)	Inhibiting tumor growth, hindering cardinogens
Polyphenols	Olive oil, berries, green tea, coffee, red wine, grapes	Antioxidants, anti-inflammatory
Ellagic acid (phenol)	Raspberries, blackberries, cranberries, strawberries, walnuts	Anti-cancer
Allyl sulfides	Garlic and onions	Anti-bacterial, may help strengthen immunity
Luteolin	Celery	Helps heal cell damage from toxicity
Saponins	Beans	Interference with DNA replication which could prevent the multiplication of cancer cells

These are three of the major phytochemical groups that can commonly be accounted for simply by eating fruits and vegetables. Though they are technically non-essential nutrients, in that our body doesn't need them, their potential benefits cannot be ignored.

Many of the best sources of phytochemicals in the diet are whole foods, which means if you're already seeking low-carbohydrate sources of vitamins and minerals, you'll find there are the added benefits of each plant's phytochemicals.

The long and short of it: the links between individual phytochemicals and the risk of disease is extremely compelling, and enough to make these nutrients a substantial part of your daily meals.

APPENDIX VI:

Maximized Metabolix for Pregnancy and Kids

When you're pregnant, you really are eating for two. While you don't need twice the calories, you do have to think twice about what you put in your system. You choices will impact two futures now.

What is Baby-weight?

In truth, there are a lot of different factors that constitute baby weight, from the actual weight of the baby to an increase in amniotic fluid—and even extra blood.

Nutrition plays a major role in pregnancy, not only in helping the mother deal with all of the energy demands placed on her body, but in ensuring that the fetal development is as healthy as possible. In this section, you'll read all about the scientific recommendations for healthy weight gain, proper nutrition, as well as how to keep children healthy as they grow into adolescence and adulthood.

Pregnancy:
Healthy Weight Gain and Getting the Right Nutrients

Because a baby depends entirely on its pregnant mother for nutrition, you know you have to pay special attention to your diet during the months of pregnancy. As is the case for any of us, too much nutrition can be just as bad as too little nutrition, which is why it's so important to understand what you're putting into your body.[257, 258, 259, 260]

Let's start with one of the biggest questions new mothers have about nutrition and pregnancy: **"How much weight should I really gain?"**

Recommendations for Weight Gain During Pregnancy

This is perhaps one of the most hotly debated topics about nutrition and pregnancy: how much actual weight should you gain throughout the pregnancy? If it seems like there is no one single answer, that's because there actually isn't.

The more you research weight gain during pregnancy, the more you realize there is no hard and fast rule that will certainly apply to your specific body type. Every woman starts out pregnancy at a different size. However, there are still some general guidelines you can use as a potential "window" for your weight gain:

General Recommendations: Weight Gain During Pregnancy[261, 262]	
Underweight women with a BMI under 19	**28–40 pounds**
Normal weight with a BMI 19–25	**25–35 pounds**

Overweight women with a BMI 25–29	15–25 pounds
Obese women with a BMI over 30	11–20 pounds

The baby will only weigh, typically, around 6–8 pounds. The rest of the weight often comes in the form of:

- 3–4 pounds of placenta and amniotic fluid
- 2–3 pounds of an enlarged uterus
- 5–8 pounds of normal extra fat
- 5–6 pounds of fluid in the tissues
- 3–4 pounds of extra blood.[263]

It's important not to gain too much weight beyond these typical numbers. Even after the "baby weight" disappears, mothers can have a tough time losing the additional weight that wasn't directly involved with the baby, or "non-baby weight." Gaining more weight than is recommended will not provide any additional benefits to the baby, but instead will simply make losing weight after the birth that much harder.

Additional Calories and Protein Required During Pregnancy

The old expression is that when you're pregnant, you're "eating for two." Nutritionally speaking, this is true! Pregnant women need more of everything: more calories, more micronutrients, more essential nutrients, more vitamin A, vitamin D, calcium, iron, iodine, EPA, DHA—the list goes on and on.

However, the need for more nutrition does not imply a need for unlimited nutrition. If you're already eating a standard diet of approximately 1,800 to 2,000 calories per day, you may only require a modest

Don't Forget Whole, Metabolix Foods

Be careful when you're eating for two. The increased need for specific nutrients is very real. Additional nutrients shouldn't come from midnight runs for ice cream and Philly cheese steaks with extra pickles—you'll go way beyond the calories necessary without getting the right nutrients. (Of course, if you're a man like me, do not question this tactic if your wife makes the request!)

increase of fifteen percent more calories. Once more, your individual requirements will vary depending on what you've already been eating.

Let's start addressing your additional nutrient needs by focusing on the "big" categories of food: total energy and macronutrients. A specific focus on protein is important in fetal development:

Total Calories: If already eating a 1,800–2,000 calorie per day diet, look to increase by approximately twelve to fifteen percent. Your maximum caloric increase should be 340 calories in the second trimester and 450 calories in the third trimester.[264]

Protein: Protein requirements can rise above RDA guidelines for women to as high as 1.1 grams per kilogram of bodyweight per day. This can mean as much as a fifty percent increase in protein intake over the low, standard guidelines. This is important for fetal growth as well as the production of breast milk.[265]

An important note: if you are already consuming fifteen to twenty-five percent of calories from protein like we recommend, on a 2,000 calorie diet, that already puts you at over seventy-five grams. At that level, there will not be a need to increase your protein.

As with other food recommendations during pregnancy, focus on quality, clean, whole proteins. And for vegetarians, your average intake of proteins tends to be low per day, so you may need to make a small additional effort to ensure you're getting adequate protein.[266]

Specific Nutrient Requirements

As you well know from reading the earlier portions of this book, calories and protein are not the only essential nutrients in the diet. In pregnancy, you will need higher amounts of a whole range of micronutrients as well. You'll recognize many of these as the same nutrients you need, but now they deserve a special focus because of the roles they play in fetal development. You already know all the nutrients your body needs to get healthier and stay healthy. Let's take a closer look at some specific nutrients that will be especially vital in maintaining your child's health.

Folate

Folate, also known as Folic acid (which is technically a kind of folate) as vitamin B9, from the appendix on vitamins. It's the water-soluble vitamin that is vital to synthesizing and repairing DNA—which, of course, gives it an important role in the growth of the fetus.

Folate deficiency can be a scary thing—it can even cause neural tube defects like spina bifida. And because these defects can form thirty days after conception and earlier, getting enough folate (at least 400 mcg per day) is important, even if you merely think you may be pregnant or are trying to get pregnant.

What's the difference between folate and folic acid? The distinction is important.

- **Folates** are B vitamins found in leafy green vegetables. Generally, when you hear the term "folate," it might refer to both folates and folic acid.

- **Folic acid** a synthetic compound that is added to vitamin-fortified foods and dietary supplements. It isn't a natural, whole nutrient, and if you take too much of it, it can reach toxic levels. So look for whole food supplements that contain folate.

Rich sources of folate that will help you in getting your daily recommended amounts: leafy green vegetables, citrus fruits, and beans. (See our soaked and sprouted section in the appendix for handling beans).

While women in pre-pregnancy, pregnancy, and breast-feeding will want to make sure they get their folate needs from a high-quality supplement, you should try to get folate from those whole foods mentioned as well. It is possible to over-do your folate supplementation, so consult with your doctor to make sure you're getting the right amount. (You'll note the "pregnant" and "lactating" suggestions at the bottom of the table.)

The recommended dietary allowances (RDAs) for folate are as follows:[267, 268]
- 600 mcg DFE when pregnant
- 500 mcg DFE when lactating

Vitamin A and Vitamin D

Vitamin A, one of the fat-soluble vitamins, certainly follows the rule of "don't get too little … or too much." A general guideline of 750 mcg/day during pregnancy and 1,200 mcg/day during lactation is usually appropriate for most mothers.[269]

Vitamin D, another of the fat-soluble vitamins, supports absorption of calcium for use in bones as well as gene programming. Without it, diseases like rheumatoid arthritis and cancer may be more likely to appear.[270, 271, 272] Getting enough vitamin D can be difficult without a supplement, which is why a recommendation of 400IU may require supplementation outside of your whole food sources.

If you're unsure about your vitamin D intake, a blood test may be in order; many sources recommend that your intake should be determined based on the levels in your blood. Consult with your doctor about vitamin D intake to be sure you're getting enough.

Common Supplements and Requirements during Pregnancy and Post-Childbirth

Thanks to its increased demand during pregnancy, one of the most common deficiencies during these months is that of iron. In fact, the need for iron is so great that it's difficult to get enough from the diet, which means it can require supplementation.

- Iron: 30mg of iron per day.[273]

Another element to pay attention to is iodine. You don't need a lot of iodine on a daily basis, but its presence is required for normal thyroid function, which helps foster the ideal physical and mental growth of the baby.[274]

It's very easy to get the small amount of iodine required. One teaspoon of iodized salt exceeds both numbers recommended below and would eliminate the need to supplement.
- Iodine: 220mcg per day for pregnant women, and 290mcg per day for breast feeding women.

Do you remember EPA and DHA from "Get an Oil Change"?
These are already crucial nutrients no matter what your pregnancy status.
They're also critical during those critical months, helping especially with vision.

In addition to being critical during pregnancy, it's important to intake EPA and DHA during breast-feeding. Considering that as much as **fifty percent** of the energy found in breast milk is in the form of fat (especially the fatty acids EPA and DHA), this should come as no surprise. Women eating plant-based diets with limited access to fish or fish oil may find that the fatty acid composition of their breast milk is not as favorable.[167] Daily supplementation of DHA also decreases the risk of the child developing food allergies and even eczema during the first year of its life.

> **EPA and DHA:** 300mg/day, although I've seen recommendations go as high as 600mg/ day. EPA and DHA are typically under-consumed in the diet. You can find EPA and DHA in the fish on the "safe list" for supplementation. Additionally, some studies have shown that maternal supplementation of AA and DHA is associated with long-term positive effects in neurodevelopment in the baby.[275, 276, 277, 278]

If that wasn't reason enough to think about EPA and DHA, consider that there have been some studies showing benefits in supplementing baby formula with these fatty acids. Unsurprisingly, the studies suggest that these can aid in visual and neural development.[279, 280]

To further foster a healthy breast-milk profile, consider making sure that you're getting enough lauric acid during the months of breastfeeding. Lauric acid's anti-microbial properties can help infants stave off illness early on. As discussed earlier on, you can find lauric acid in coconut oil.

A Note on Fish for Pregnant Women

If you're eating fish to add protein, EPA, and DHA to your diet, then, as a pregnant woman, you'll really want to pay attention to the list of clean fish that are lower in mercury than their high-mercury counter parts. Refer to the list of low-mercury fish in "iProtein" to make sure you get EPA and DHA from safe sources while pregnant.

Post-Pregnancy and Beyond:
Proper Nutrition for Growing Kids

After the baby is born, you're no longer "eating for two," but that doesn't mean you're any less concerned with the nutrition your child receives. Quite the opposite: now, perhaps more than any time in your child's life, quality nutrition is of vital importance.

These parenting instincts are confirmed by the science: there are many studies that show that proper nutrition in the first year of your child's life can have positive effects that last into adulthood. If you want your baby to grow into a healthy, happy child and ultimately a healthy, happy adult, it starts in those first months, and it starts with breast-feeding.

Breast Milk: Nature's Best Baby Food

As a mother, your body has been provided the means to offer your newly-born child one of the best possible whole foods there is: breast milk. There are reasons that breast milk comes packed with a specific formula of nutrients; they're good for your baby!

There's a reason your doctors want you to breast-feed. Breast-feeding is incredibly important to the growth, development, and overall wellbeing of your child. Consider all of the areas of health and wellness that natural breast milk has to offer your newborn:

The Health Benefits of Breast Feeding

Benefits	Source
Breastfeeding exclusively until six months and partially until twelve months provides optimal nutrition for babies.	Position of the American Dietetic Association, Journal of the American Dietetic Association, 2009[281]
If U.S. breastfeeding rates were raised, less infant deaths may result.	Pediatrics[282]
Potential prevention of childhood leukemia.	Journal of the National Cancer Institute, 1999[283]
Reduced risk of cancer.	Medical & Pediatric Oncology, 1991[284]
Prevention of rheumatoid arthritis—even into adulthood.	British Medical Journal, 2003[285]
Lower rates of ear infections.	Pediatri Infect Dis J, 1994[286]
Higher IQ.	Journal of the American Medical Association, 2002[287]
Higher cognitive scores.	American Journal of Clinical Nutrition, 1999[288]
Prevention of respiratory illness.	Archives of Disease in Childhood, 2003[289]
Reduction in respiratory tract illnesses.	Archives of Pediatrics and Adolescent Medicine, 2003[290]
Prevention of diarrhea.	The Pediatric Infectious Disease Journal, 1994[291]
Prevention of asthma.	British Medical Journal, 1999[292]
Prevention of diabetes.	Diabetes Care, 1998[293]

In short, if you want your baby to have the healthiest possible beginning to their life, you'll want to make sure they're breast-fed well and often.

But don't forget that breast-feeding helps you, as well! Many studies have shown that women who breast-feed have lower risks of developing breast cancer.[294, 295, 296]

Food for babies to avoid

Avoid commercial (not organic), grain-fed cow's milk, as well as eggs, seafood, nuts, corn, soy, soy formulas, wheat, caffeine, fruit drinks, and soft drinks.

Children and Adolescence

Of course, you can't feed your child breast milk all their life. Eventually, you'll wean your child off of breast milk and onto other foods—and soon, breast milk won't even be part of their diet.

The principles of nutrition as you've read them throughout this book begin to come into play here. Rather than ensuring good nutrition for yourself and giving your child breast milk, you now have to make other choices for your child as they grow into adolescence.

Protein

As protein plays a critical role in growth, children may need slightly more protein than does the average adult. Since the goal is to start feeding your infant food outside of breast milk (though still including breast milk) somewhere between six months and a year, that's where the nutrition recommendations begin.

Protein With Little Meat

It's possible, even for kids. Although the best sources of protein are meat, there are plenty of other ways for children to get protein, including from nuts, seeds, nut/seed butters, vegetables, and even a moderate amount of non-gluten, non-GMO grains.[357]

Once again, RDAs for protein are low; Children ages one to three is 13g; four to eight is 19g; nine to thirteen is 34g; fourteen to eighteen is 46g for a girl, and 52g for a boy. The average kids are likely eating more than that.[297, 298] The Maximized Metabolix recommendations will again be as a percentage of total calories and above standards, without being "high protein." For children, this is twenty to twenty-five percent of their total calories and looking to be in the 15-25g/meal range.

Total Calories for Adolescents

Kids' and adolescents' diets tend to be calorie-dense rather than nutrient-dense. Chips, fries, candy, and sodas are the norm—when the focus should be on vegetables, fruits, meats, and whole foods.

How many daily calories should your child be getting as they grow up? It depends on a number of factors, including size and activity level. An *Institute of Medicine Dietary Reference Intakes* report in 2002 put together the following table:

Gender	Age (years)	Sedentary	Moderately Active	Active
Child	2–3	1,000	1,000–1,400	1,000–1,400
Female	4–8	1,200	1,400–1,600	1,400–1,800
	9–13	1,600	1,600–2,000	1,800–2,200
	14–18	1,800	2,000	2,400
Male	4–8	1,400	1,400–1,600	1,600–2,000
	9–13	1,800	1,800–2,200	2,000–2,600
	14–18	2,200	2,400–2,800	2,800–3,200

299

Because the caloric intake is separated by your child's activity level, note the definitions of each category:

Sedentary: The only physical activity is that which is required to go about a daily routine—walking around, picking up objects, etc. In a sedentary lifestyle, no extra exercise or activity is offered.

Moderately active: On top of the activity required in daily life, a moderately active lifestyle includes the extra exercise equivalent of walking one-and-a-half to two miles per day.

Active: Same as above, except now the additional activity level exceeds the equivalent of walking three miles per day.

As a parent, you'll have a good idea of your child's activity level, so this chart should serve as a handy reference. But remember that it's merely a guide, not a limit. Each child is different, and you should make sure yours has enough energy to function throughout the day.

Example Protein Requirements for Children:
Protein is Twenty to Twenty-five Percent of Calories

For more help, utilize the Protein and Carb counters in **Chapter Seven**.

Example 1: 1000–1,400 Calories, 50g–88g of Protein
2 eggs = 16g
3 oz. of chicken breast = 24g
4 oz. hamburger = 28g
TOTAL = 68g

Example 2: 1,400–1,800 Calories, 70g–113g of Protein
Grass-fed whey protein smoothie with chia seeds = 29g1/4 cup of almonds = 8g
4oz salmon = 24g
4oz steak = 28g
Yogurt = 10g
TOTAL = 99g

Vegetarian Example 3: 1,600–2,000 Calories, 80g–125g of Protein
Sprouted vegetable protein smoothie with flax seeds = 28g
2 Tbsp of almond butter = 14g
1 cup of beans = 20g 1/2 cup of cashews = 10g
Salad with chia, flax, and garbanzo beans = 32g
TOTAL = 104g

Example 4: 2,400–2,800 Calories, 120–175g of Protein

4 eggs with cheese = 30g

1/2 cup of almonds = 16g

4 oz of chicken = 32g

6 oz steak = 42g

Grass-fed whey smoothie = 25g

TOTAL = 145g

APPENDIX VII:

Exercise and Sports
Training Low

The Recommendations for the Best Athletes in the World—And You

Sports are what got me and many of our doctors into nutrition in the first place. As much as any other area, performance is a passion—which is why I get so bothered by the processed food approach many athletes and athletic programs take.

Rule #1 is pretty simple: athletes should avoid the many "health and fitness" powders, bars, and snacks that contain refined sugars, processed proteins, inorganic, and artificial ingredients, additives, and preservatives. All of these create the poor health we've been talking about, can cause injury, and certainly hinder the results competitors are striving towards.

Some athletes seem to get away with eating junk. The reason is some combination of carb tolerance and the fact that hard training and competition can help alleviate some of the dangers and inflammatory effects of sugars and grains. But this approach catches up with everybody. You just can't eat poorly and avoid injury, create health and longevity, and perform at your greatest potential.

Good Training Starts with Good Nutrition

Whether you are gifted with athletic ability or not, the right nutrition can make all the difference in the results you get from your training and exercise. Many of the professional and Olympic athletes we've worked with know that nutrition can ultimately be the difference between winning and losing.

How to Maximize Your Exercise Without Excess Carbohydrates

My wife and I do endurance sports as a hobby. I know—most of you are probably saying, "Really? Fun hobby. Have you tried scuba diving or backgammon?"

But we love it. Not only are endurance sports social, but they help keep us fit as we make our way deep into our upper forties. From Olympic distance

Training low

Training Low is the term for keeping sugar low in your fitness routine, and it's particularly helpful if your goals include retaining lean mass, cutting fat, and radically improving your hormone function. It's especially important for those with a tendency to put on fat tissue.

triathlons to half- and full-marathons, we make an effort to think about our blood glucose and our body's glycogen stores. At these extreme distances, carbs are often necessary.

Before long training or a multi-hour event, we put berries in a smoothie to ensure that our glycogen is where it needs to be. Berries are whole foods, with anti-oxidant and anti-inflammatory properties, so we know we're getting our carbohydrates from a healthy, low glycemic source. We're also getting some fuel to help our bodies deal with the side-effects of endurance exercise without suffering the consequences of refined, processed carbohydrates.

During and after training lasting more than an hour, coconut water is the preferred drink over "sports drinks." As I'll share later on, coconut water can help meet most of your training needs without all the adulterations of processed recovery drinks. So-called "sports drinks" are often made palatable by a high concentration of sugar, which has a glucose replacing effect—but that only helps you if you have glucose to replace. During long, intense activities, this might be a consideration, particularly if you train in a place like Florida, where it's brutally hot and humid most of the year.

Most people, however, aren't training that long or under those conditions, so do not require anything for recovery.

I also work with professional and Olympic athletes, many of whom train two–three times per day, for hours on end. When you train that often, you may need to think about glycogen stores and keeping them stocked.

But even in these extreme circumstances, are processed power bars and neon green, blue, and yellow, sugary recovery products a good way to go? The ultimate, long-term hurt likely far outweighs any short-term help.

Wherever you find your training needs, look to whole foods first.

When it comes to sugar-replacement, unless it's marathon day or you're at a training camp and working out multiple times a day while vying for a spot in professional sports, you'll have little need to increase sugar.

Training low, without all of the sugar, is the way to go for the vast majority of people. Again, look to burn fats rather than carbs. In fact, not only can you train low, but it's the best way to achieve the healthy, lean body you're exercising to get in the first place.

Aerobic vs. Anaerobic Exercise

There are essentially three "modes" in which your body burns energy. Much of it hinges on a concept known as "VO2 Max," or your body's maximum level of oxygen consumption. Your VO2 Max level is individual to you.

Activity Level	Description
Resting	The most common form of activity today! In resting, your muscles prefer fat for fuel. You'll actually burn most of your calories this way, since most of our time is spent sitting, sleeping, or remaining relatively inactive. You want to burn fat while resting.
Aerobic Exercise	Usually defined as exercise somewhere below 60% of your VO2 Max, aerobic exercise refers to exercise "with air." You can still carry a conversation in aerobic exercise, which means you're getting enough air to sustain the activity for a while.
Anaerobic exercise (High intensity, short duration MaxT3 type)	Exercise "without air," this generally refers to exercise greater than 70% of VO2 Max. You'll be exercising so hard at this point that you'll continue "sucking in air" even after you finish. This is your body making up for the lack of oxygen during the exercise yourself. As you'll see later, this type of exercise can be very effective for fat loss.

Over-Rated, Misunderstood Sugar

When it comes to the world of fitness, sugar may be the most overrated substance there is. Even in the presence of exercise, the basic rules of food and understanding its impact on your physiology still apply.

You'd be surprised how pervasive these nutritional misunderstandings are. In preparation for the 2012 Olympics, we worked with the US weightlifting team. I went as one of their doctors to the US Championships in Peoria, Illinois. Throughout my time with them, I saw Olympic-class weightlifters drinking Powerade and Gatorade and indulging in fried-chicken sandwiches on white bread.

I was astounded. Sure, if you're in the second hour of a marathon, then your body probably needs glucose. If you're running a 10k or even working out intensely for a several minutes, you could argue for the need of carbohydrates in your system.

But as a weightlifter, eating this way can only hurt your performance and sap your strength. In fact, in just a few seconds, I can show you how sugar can dramatically hinder your athletic performance. It's something I've done hundreds of times when speaking, with everyone from amateur to Olympic-level and professional athletes.

Here's how it works: grab anyone in your home, have them hold their arm out and try to push their arm down as they resist. Note their strength. With elite, strength-trained athletes, you won't be able to push their arm down. You might even be able to do some pull-ups off of their arms.

Next, have them put half-a-teaspoon of sugar in their mouth and retest their arm strength. Their arm will practically flop down.

Sugar is an anti-nutrient. It's "kryptonite" to athletic performance. The idea that sugar is needed for any type of performance beyond solving glucose and glycogen depletion in endurance and intense, multi-hour training is simply wrong.

That's why trying to make an Olympic team while loading up on sugar-heavy "sports drinks" is a good way to find yourself watching the event from home. Not only is the sugar unnecessary, but it is actively hindering your attempts to reach your goals.

This leaves us with some very important questions: how do you best fuel your body when you're working out? How can you stay at your best when in the throes of athletic competition? How can you exercise without setting off all of the inflammatory, aging, and weight-gaining principles behind carbohydrates in the diet?

The answers to all of these questions rest on a number of factors, including:

- Type of exercise
- How often you exercise
- Your personal fitness goals
- The intensity of your exercise

Once you grasp the principles of training low, you'll begin to see how nutrition can work to keep your body moving towards your health goals.

High Intensity Training for Athletes while Training Low

The science of burning fat during periods of high-intensity performance is still young, but there are several good studies that show that if you can adapt your body to burning fat, you can increase performance without having to switch to sugar-burning, right away. This is done through switching from a sugar burner to a fat burner, like we showed you in the Carbs chapter. The Advanced plan focuses on fat for fuel. Additionally, for active athletes and exercisers, the low end of the Core Plan, taking in 75–125g of carbs a day, is also relying a whole lot on fat energy.

Some of the findings in these studies point to the possibility that our utilization of sugar for fuel may be due to the fact that our bodies are not "fat-adapted."

A 1994 study found that those high-intensity exercisers who were fed a high-fat diet showed a greater resistance to fatigue while making sparing use of the carbohydrates in the diet.[300] A 1996 study concluded that "the short-term ketogenic diet does not impair aerobic exercise capacity…" It even increased VO2 max![301] And a study in Metabolism found that athletes in ketosis did not suffer from impaired athletic performance.[302]

What are we left to conclude? Well, these are just three studies, but the science seems to suggest that switching from carbohydrate burning to fat burning does not impede performance. In some cases, it may even enhance it.

Sucking Air and Burning Fat After Exercise

When most people think about burning energy for exercise, they just think about what's going on during their effort. "If I need short-term energy," they figure, "then what better than carbs and sugar?"

EPOC

Excess Post-exercise Oxygen Consumption is the lasting energy effect created every single time you exercise. It's most triggered during more intense, anaerobic exercise.

But there's a secondary need for fuel even after the exercise is over. When your exercise intensity is high, not only will you burn sugar and/or fat during your workout, but you will continue to burn energy throughout the rest of the day.

This is known as **EPOC: Excess Post-exercise Oxygen Consumption**. You might call it "breathing hard." Even after your physical effort has ended, your body still has metabolic needs. If you do a high-intensity sprint or a set of burpees, while the exercise is considered "anaerobic," or "without air," you'll still have an oxygen need after the exercise is completed. This secondary effect becomes "aerobic," or "with air" metabolism.[303, 304, 305, 306, 307] Thus, the heavy breathing.

The higher the intensity of your exercise, the greater the EPOC effect. At this point, if you hit the right intensity threshold, you'll end up using fat for fuel.[308,]

The Fat-Burning Department

When fat is broken down and "burned" in your body, it's done so through the process of lipolysis and beta-oxidation. These reactions occur in what might be considered your body's "fat-burning department," the mitochondria. Because they burn your body's best source of fuel, the mitochondria are the energy warehouses of the cells.

The process is cyclical. Two carbon atoms are removed from long fatty acid chains, helping form a molecule known as acetyl-CoA. This molecule will enter the citric acid cycle to produce energy in the form of ATP. This process uses an identical pathway for glucose molecules when they are used for energy rather than being stored as fat.

Mitochondria "feed" energy to your muscles by converting food to ATP energy using the same process you just read about. Fat loss happens when fatty acids are removed from their storage, where you don't want it, and given to mitochondria to be oxidized and burned for their energy.

Needless to say, mitochondria are very important. The good news is that you can actually increase not only the effectiveness of these mitochondria, but their number. You accomplish this through exercise. (Of course, maybe you wouldn't consider that good news, depending on how you feel about exercise.) Ultimately, the more you exercise, the more efficient and effective your body will be at burning fat.

If you had access to money-printing machines, you'd want as many of them as possible. So it is with burning fat: the more mitochondria you have, the more efficient they are, and the better off you'll be. By increasing the number of mitochondria, you increase "mitochondrial density." This density allows the mitochondria to do a better, more efficient job at changing over the fat into ATP so you can get lean. Your body will burn fat more efficiently, and you'll use your energy for muscles rather than storage.

The question, then, is how do you create more mitochondria—a process known as mitochondrial biogenesis—and increase their density as well?

You do it through exercise, including high-intensity training, lower-intensity endurance training, and resistance training, or weight training.[309, 310 311, 312]

The more difficult and consistent your training is, the more your body will need to create mitochondria.

Conclusion
Switch from sugar burning to fat burning and add mitochondria, and you are one serious fat-burning force to be reckoned with.

MaxT3 to Max Out The Fat Burning Benefits of Exercise

While traditional cardiovascular exercise like jogging on a treadmill or cycling does burn calories, the length of time required to complete such a workout can actually have negative effects.

This long-duration, low-intensity exercise can actually cause the body to begin storing calories as fat, as it triggers the production of the catabolic stress hormones and does little to maximize the good anabolic hormones.

On the contrary, programs like Max T3 use short-duration, high-intensity exercise. This type of workout requires short bursts of maximum to near-maximum effort. This boosts fat-burning, muscle-building hormones and increases the resting metabolic rate via the "afterburner effect"—which is the excess post-exercise oxygen consumption (EPOC), explained earlier.

This effect improves your physiology and encourages the body to continue burning fat and calories for up to two full days after a workout has been completed.

The three "Ts" in Max T3 are Time, Tempo, and Type. By shortening the time, increasing the tempo effort, and using more multi-joint types of exercise, you'll get the full impact of Maximized Metabolix.

Getting the Best Bang for Your Workout Buck

"I work out, I work out, and I work out, and still I don't seem to lose any weight."
Have you ever met someone like this? Have you ever been this person? If you've been working out and not seeing any fat loss for your efforts, it may be because you're eating far too many carbs—certainly more than your body needs.

Most people who exercise are looking to eliminate body fat, or what essentially equates to "stored carbs in the form of fat."

If you eat too many carbs, you'll burn them rather than the sugar and fat energy stores already present in your body.

For those of you who don't see a lot of fat loss as a result of working out consistently, it might be because you're not training low. In other words, your diet is providing all of the energy you need to exercise, which means you don't have to tap your stored fat to get through the workouts and refuel your body afterwards.

When energy balance is maintained, your exercise will not induce a negative fat balance. Although endurance training does increase the capacity of your muscle mitochondria to utilize your fat as fuel, carbohydrates can change the game from fat to sugar.

When carbohydrates are consumed, a rise in insulin follows. As a result, lipolysis (breaking down of fat for fuel) is suppressed by the presence of insulin.

Even tiny amounts of glucose or fructose have been shown to suppress your body's ability to burn fat even after waiting one hour before the start of exercise.[313] If eating carbohydrates essentially turns off your body's ability to burn fat, it will clash directly with your fat loss goals, neutralizing all of your hard work. If you want to get the most bang for your exercise buck, train low.

Training Low:
What You Need to Know
about Metabolics Training

Thinking Carbohydrate and Athletic Performance

What is the goal of exercise? For most people, it's to retain lean mass or grow lean mass while losing fat mass.

In order to support this goal, we recommend that you train low. If you're an athlete training at an elite level, you may want to use carbohydrates for fuel, but we still recommend whole, lower-GI (Glycemic Index) sources of carbohydrates.

A typical recommendation is to consume thirty–sixty grams of carbohydrates for every hour of exercise, if going for over an hour. We often recommend cutting back to less than forty percent of that number, or twelve–twenty-four grams of carbohydrate per every hour of exercise. Staying away from sugar, refined grains, and other high-GI foods is critical here.

Another concern when training low: muscle loss. But by engaging in resistance exercise and adding protein during a hypoenergetic (training low) dieting period, athletes will also provide the stimulus needed to retain muscle. Let's look at two examples and see what you can do to improve your ability to burn fat rather than the sugar you just ate for exercise.

The Failure of the
High–Carb Cyclist

We have many patients that are cyclists. A common scenario is that they are riding their bike in order to promote fat loss and weight loss. However, they don't end up losing a gram. If your nutrition program lines up perfectly with your workout regimen, your hard work on the bike should coincide with the burning of some body fat during the workout.

Training Low and Pre-workout Meals

A study in *Endocrinology and Metabolism*[358] in 1997 found that exercise preceded by a carbohydrate-rich meal reduced the rate of fat-burning. If you want to burn fat, make sure that you're training low.

Unfortunately, there is a common problem: the patient eats a large bowl of oatmeal, with raisins and milk, an hour prior to exercise. Insulin levels then rise to store and utilize glucose while suppressing lipolysis (fat-burning) during exercise.

As a result, while the patients sweat and suck air in and out while putting in the miles, their bodies have quite literally have turned off their own fat-burning mechanisms.

What you eat before you exercise has a dramatic effect on what happens to your energy during the workout. Some research has even indicated that at least six hours of fasting are necessary after consuming five to six hundred calories in carbohydrates before you can move past "sugar-burning" during your workout.[314]

Switching Your Pre-Workout Meals

If you work out hard and don't burn any fat, it's likely you just burn the sugar you eat instead of cashing in on any of your fuel reserves.

In order to burn fat during exercise, your insulin levels will need to be low. Because carbohydrates stimulate insulin the most out of any macronutrient, you need to be wary about when you eat them, and in what quantities.

Sugar taken in pre-exercise will also impede HGH—human growth hormone. This is a good hormone, needed to build muscle and burn fat.

Why Exercise in the Morning?

Working out first thing in the morning on an empty stomach offers a number of benefits, including:

- Best compliance—you won't procrastinate all day.
- Raised growth hormone.
- Highest testosterone impact.
- Insulin is low, aiding with fat burning.
- "Charging" your metabolism and feel good hormones for the day.

In the morning (after an overnight "fast"), your insulin levels will be low. The mornings are therefore a great time to work out.

But, if you want to maximize your fat burning during the morning workout, you should limit your carbohydrate level at breakfast to eight grams or less—or even skip breakfast altogether.

So what should you eat in a pre-exercise meal if you want to be sure you're not hungry, but you do want to maximize fat burning? Here are four sample meals you can put together that will fill you up, give you plenty of flavor, but won't stuff you full of fat cell-suppressing carbohydrates:

Pre-Exercise Meals to Maximize Fat Burning

Breakfast 1:	Grass-fed whey smoothie with stevia and 2 oz. of coconut milk
Breakfast 2:	3/4 cup cottage cheese and 2 Tbsp. blueberries
Breakfast 3:	3-egg white omelet with 1/2 diced tomato and 2 Tbsp. onion
Snack:	Green apple or celery with tbsp. of almond butter
Lunch 1:	Lettuce turkey wrap, including tomato and 3 oz. sliced, nitrate-free turkey

Lunch 2:	1 cup Greek or goat's milk yogurt, plain, with stevia and shaved, unsweetened chocolate

Note that these meals don't actually include a whole lot of fat. Why not? As it turns out, a high-fat meal consumed close to exercise can impede the release of the very growth hormones you want working in order to retain lean mass.[315]

Post-Workout Meals and the "Magic Window"

Many people focus on what they eat before a workout, but don't really take the time to consider what they should eat after a workout. If you've had a particularly taxing workout that does require some carbohydrates in order for your body to recover, there's a one-hour "magic window" in which you should consume some food to ensure the best effects.

With your muscles eating up energy, the first sixty minutes after exercise can help you "put away" carbs in the least harmful fashion. Note that you don't want to consume sugary sports drinks and sweetened sports bars.

Just like before a workout, high doses of glucose following a workout will undermine a lot of what you're trying to accomplish by impeding good, fat-burning, muscle-building growth hormone released during and after exercise.

A good recovery meal ratio is **1:1 carbs:protein** which will include twenty–twenty-five grams of protein and twenty–twenty-five grams of carbohydrate. This is a good "synergy" meal that will help you recover from a long bout of exercise. An organic, unpasteurized, grass-fed whey protein powder is highly bioavailable to meet protein needs. Combined this with low glycemic-index berries in a smoothie, and you will make sure you don't get the big blood-sugar spike and hinder the better body hormones you're looking to leverage.

Timing Your Protein Just Right
You can maximize the effects of protein comes to protein by timing it correctly. Studies show that timing your protein after exercise can be very important.[316, 317]

One study in the *Journal of Physiology*[318] concluded that taking in protein immediately after resistance training helped elderly subjects experience the hypertrophy, or muscle-building, that they desired.

A 2011 study found that consuming protein after exercise was associated with increased "de novo muscle protein synthesis," which means new muscle proteins were created.[319]

A 2004 study found that taking in whey proteins in particular helped build muscle after resistance exercise.[320]

Other data has shown that rather than simply timing your protein right after exercise, the most important thing is that you have enough protein in your system to deal with the tissue breakdown that occurs through exercise.

Keto-Adapted Exercise

As you read previously, extreme carbohydrate limitation will leave you in ketosis, or "keto-adapted" after as little as a few weeks. For those who are very sensitive to carbs, this disciplined approach can be effective at controlling insulin, blood sugar, and ensuring that you're burning fat full-time.

Since the brain can only run on either glucose, ketones, or some combination of the two, it has to rely on these fuels to get by. There is no glycogen supply present in the brain, as there is in skeletal muscles and your liver. That means your brain relies on the blood to get its fuel, which is why a drop in blood sugar can lead to brain problems, such as sinking into a coma. Does this mean you can't exercise while in ketosis? Of course not. If your brain is running on ketones and the available whole foods carbs you're eating, it's getting along just fine.

Many of our doctors and patients don't do many carbs. With our focus on berries in the morning, coconut products, vegetables, fats, and proteins—it just doesn't add up much more beyond the ketogenic level. Yet, we can work out very long and hard, all the while burning fats.

Long Distance Training
Good News

During exercise, as blood glucose levels fall, so do insulin levels. This is perfectly fine if your exercise is somewhat limited, or even if it's somewhat difficult but you still aren't exercising as much as an endurance or professional athlete.

But what if you are exercising that much? For long endurance training and elites doing multiple daily workouts, you may need glucose replenishment.

In some cases, you can eat carbohydrates for glucose replenishment without the associated insulin effects.

During a workout, if muscle contraction is serving as a stimulus for transportation of glucose into the muscle cell, then glucose is taken out of the blood stream before it has its effect on insulin. As a result, a carbohydrate supplement consumed during exercise will not cause the wild spike in insulin it otherwise would cause. The associated inflammation, insulin resistance, and suppression of fat oxidation that all come with increased insulin would be neutralized.[321]

From Grandmas to Little League to the Olympics and the Pros
What You Need to Know

No matter who you are, there are three major rules to healthy sports nutrition that will keep you healthy, lean, and ultimately provide you the best path to quick recovery:

1

The Whole Food Rule

Keep it clean. Back to this tenet of Maximized Metabolics. Processed carbs, drinks, drugs, supplements—they're simply the wrong way to go about keeping your body fueled. Even if they appear to pay off in the short term, you can sacrifice your future health; in essence, you're robbing Peter to pay Paul. It comes down to this: you can't fool mother nature. The synergy of nutrients in a "whole food" system of eating simply cannot be found in a bottle. Sure, sports supplements can enhance performance, but for long-term health and training, you can't beat the God-given balance found in whole, natural foods.

2

For the Very Active, "Carb Consciousness" may not be as High a Priority

For the very active, "carb consciousness" may not be as high a priority. If weight loss is not your goal and your carb tolerance is high, you may not have to worry about taking in so many carbs. This isn't a free pass to eat carbs with lots of sugar and grains (and breaking Rule #1), as they can exacerbate inflammation, injury, and poor performance problems and lead to long-term consequences you don't want to deal with.

3

Training low is the way to go

Training low is the way to go. Unless you're an extreme endurance athlete exercising multiple hours a day or training for the big race, you won't have to worry so much about recovery. A healthy, whole diet will easily replace glycogen stores, and a moderate increase of protein will help you retain lean mass. When you train low, you rip through your fat stores, which in turn helps meet your weight-loss goals. Once your body adapts to burning more fat, you'll become more efficient at using fat for energy. As a result, your performance can ultimately improve without the side-effects of inflammation to hamper your physical training.

Athletes should avoid typical processed foods. Many "health and fitness" snacks contain refined sugars, artificial ingredients, additives, and preservatives that create poor health, increase the chance of injury, and can hinder the results competitors are looking for.

Hard training and competition can help alleviate some of the dangers and inflammatory effects of sugars and grains. But it's hardly something to focus your meal planning around in order to avoid injury, create health and longevity, and perform at your greatest potential.

Some packaged fitness snacks use natural sugars and contain no chemical additives. While high sugar is rarely a great training-table suggestion, athletes training for multiple hours or multiple times a day may benefit in recovery from glucose replenishing foods and drinks.

The following are foods to **avoid for training**:

Simple Meal/Snack Items

• Granola and sports bars	• Commercial crackers and chips—trans fats and chemicals
• Sports recovery drinks	• Bagels and breads—additives, preservatives, gluten, refined grains, and very high glycemic index
• Commercial peanut butter, other nut butters, and jelly	• Commercial cereal—chemicals, additives, preservatives, sugars, refined grains, and gluten
• Powdered meal supplement	• Instant rice—no fiber, very high glycemic index
• Tuna—it's on the high mercury list	• Instant potatoes—higher GI than candy bar or table sugar
• Commercial beef jerky—filled with MSG	• Instant breakfast drinks—high sugar and artificial ingredients
• Chicken, beef pouches—artificial ingredients	• Soy powders and ingredients
• Instant noodles, ramen noodles—chemical seasonings	

The following is the **on-the-go** food list we prepared for several of the United States teams to use as they prepare and travel to events like the World Cup, World Championships, and Olympics:

Travel Snacks

• Whey concentrate protein powder	• Whole grain, gluten-free crackers
• Unsalted/unroasted nuts (preferably raw)—almonds, cashews, pistachios, walnuts	• Beef jerky has to be from a health food store; others have sulfites, nitrites, and MSG

• Fruit leather bars	• Multigrain, organic, gluten-free bagels—ideally sprouted
• Dried fruits—apples, raisins, cranberries, prunes (look out for added sugars, and try to avoid sulfites if possible)	• Green super-food powders
• Low glycemic fruit—green apples, fresh apricots, blackberries, grapefruit	• Raw dark chocolate, minimum 70% cacao content
• Trail mix—almonds, pecans, dried fruit, and sunflower seeds	• Goji berries
• Raw almond and/or peanut butter, raw honey, fruit-sweetened jam	

Protein - Eat organic whenever possible

• Packaged sardines	• Organic, no sugar or oil added almond or peanut butter
• Lean chicken breast	• Milk—coconut, almond,
• Beef, wild game	• Unsalted/unroasted nuts
• Salmon	• Whey concentrate protein powder
• Eggs	

Carbohydrate

• Vegetables	• Granola/dry cereal—organic, natural, no hydrogenated oils; best is to follow the recipe to make your own
• Berries, Granny Smith apples	• Organic, gluten-free snack crackers
• Brown rice	• Oats, oatmeal—gluten-free is best
• Lentils	• Dried fruit without added sugars or sulfites
• Spinach	• Raw, organic honey

Fat

• Olive oil	• Raw butter
• Coconut oil	• Fish oil supplement
• Sesame oil	• Flax and chia seeds—add to everything possible!

For Training With Weight Loss

We use this one for our wrestlers and professional MMA fighters.

Avanced Plan Leading up to the Event

Breakfast choices

1. Smoothie
   - 1 scoop Maximized Living Perfect Protein Powder (chocolate or vanilla)
   - 5 frozen strawberries1/2 of an avocado
   - Tbsp of chia seeds1/2 cup unsweetened coconut milk
   - 1 tbsp almond butter
   - Stevia to taste
   - (Make it green with some kale, cucumber, and/or celery)
2. Eggs and berries
3. Kitchen Sink Yogurt*
4. Ricotta or cottage cheese—Kitchen-Sink style, with berries, or plain

Pre-workout

1. Smoothie with powder, stevia, unsweetened cocoa powder, coconut milk
2. Fruit, fruit salad; low-glycemic fruits—green apples, berries, grapefruit
3. Almond butter and celery or green apple
4. Couple of handfuls of raw nuts

After workout

1. Intense, greater than one hour: one–two cups of coconut water
2. Good recovery meal ratio: 25 grams of protein, 25 gram carbohydrate is the optimal synergy meal.
   - An organic, un-pasteurized, grass-fed whey protein powder w/ fruit and coconut milk smoothie is an easy way to accomplish this ratio, or
   - Chicken, beef, or fish w/vegetables and small sweet potato

Snacks and Dessert examples (see more from our recipe list)

- Cinnamon Nut Mix
- Grainless Granola
- Almond butter and celery or green apple
- Avocado Pudding*
- Smoothie with avocado, unsweetened cocoa powder, chia seeds, stevia, and water

Dinner

1. Animal protein, vegetable, and salad recipe
2. Snack or grain-free, stevia-sweetened dessert

*See recipes

For Training Without Weight Loss—Core Plan

Breakfast choices

Add bananas, sweet potatoes, brown rice, and gluten-free grains and snacks after breakfast and lunch. Can do low-glycemic fruits and dairy products in the evening.

1. Oat meal (2 Servings), 2–4 eggs, berries, coconut or unsweetened almond milk, 1–2 Tbsp almond butter
2. 2 slices of sprouted toast, like Ezekial bread, 4 eggs, 1–2 pcs/fruit

Pre-workout

1. Berry, coconut milk, stevia, and grass-fed whey protein powder smoothie

Lunch

1. 6 oz Chicken breast, ground beef, or fish side salad,
2. brown rice or
3. sweet potato w/coconut oil

Snacks and Dessert examples (see more from our recipe list)

1. Protein shake w/ fruit, coconut water
2. Raw trail mix

Dinner

1. Steak, salad, and vegetables.

Snacks

1. 2 servings, full-fat cottage cheese
2. Protein shake
3. Almond butter on a green apple
4. Grain-free, stevia- or xylitol-sweetened dessert recipe
5. Avocado Pudding*

*See recipes

2,400 Calories for Competitive Athletes

Breakfast choices

1. Berry Smoothie*
2. Apple with 2 Tbsp almond butter
3. Water

Lunch

1. Stuffed Pepper*
2. 1 cup raspberries with 1 Tbsp sour cream
3. Water

Snacks

1. Cinnamon Almonds*

Dinner

1. 6 oz roast beef
2. 1 cup mashed sweet potatoes with 1 Tbsp coconut oil and 1/2 tsp cinnamon
3. 2 cups Brussels sprouts roasted with 1 1/2 Tbsp olive oil
4. 1 cup organic whole milk Greek or goat's milk yogurt, ground flax seeds, shaved unsweetened chocolate, with stevia or xylitol and vanilla
5. Water

*See recipes

2,600 Calories for Competitive Athletes

Breakfast choices

1. Three-egg Spanish omelet with 1 oz organic cheddar cheese, 1/4 cup salsa, and 1 cup green chilis cooked in 1 Tbsp olive oil
2. 1 cup blueberries with 1/3 cup organic sour cream
3. Water

Lunch

1. 5 oz cooked chicken breast mixed with 1/2 cup guacamole
2. Green salad and 1 cup green beans sautéed in 1 Tbsp olive oil
3. Water

Snacks

1. Chocolate Almond Butter Fudge*

Dinner

1. Salmon in Basil Cream Sauce*
2. 2 cups baked acorn squash with 1 Tbsp raw, grass-fed butter and 1 tsp pumpkin pie spice
3. 1 cup cucumbers and 1 cup cherry tomatoes with 1 Tbsp olive oil and 1 tsp balsamic vinegar
4. 1 cup strawberries
5. Water
6. Green smoothie*

*See recipes

Hydrating and Refueling the Metabolix Way

Hydration and Rehydration Recovery Drinks

The standard rule of thumb for carbohydrates and hydration during exercise, as indicated by the International Society of Sports Nutrition[322], are as follows:

Coconut Water: Nature's Sports Drink

If you want a whole, natural source for replenishing your body's fluids, try coconut water. In addition to replenishing your electrolytes, it was shown to have more favorable effects on your stomach, such as less nausea—which can be critical if you're running a race. If you can find it straight from the coconut, even better.

- Consume 30–60g of carbohydrates per hour in a 6–8% carbohydrate-water solution.
- Drink eight to sixteen ounces every ten to fifteen minutes.

Do you really need all that sugar along with your hydration?

Human beings were re-hydrating themselves long before sports drinks. It's possible for you to do the same without the massive intake of sugar associated with drinking many of these concoctions.

Here are a few tips for re-hydrating without the packaged re-hydration drinks:

- Try coconut water first. Coconut water has much less sugar and fewer calories than typical sports drinks. You might consider it "nature's sports drink." It doesn't have as much sodium as others, but it does contain more potassium, which is also an electrolyte. Coconut water is "isotonic"—it has a synergy of nutrients designed to replenish without near the negative glycemic effect of packaged sports drinks.

One study showed that coconut water will replenish your bodily fluids as well as any sports drink[323], while others pointed out that it led to less nausea and upset stomachs and was easier to consume in larger amounts.[324, 325] One word of warning: some coconut water brands add MSG to their product, so be on the lookout for those.

- Look to whole food sources. Before you drink sugar water, you can make your own fruit smoothie to get carbohydrates from a natural source that comes packed with other good stuff like fiber. You can even consume mineral-rich vegetables to replenish your electrolytes, and what's more, you'll get the associated benefits of consuming these foods.

- Avoid the sugary sports drinks. Rule of thumb? If you can buy it in a bottle at a gas station, then it might not be what's best for you. Unless, of course, you have a really good gas station in your area. But if your sports-hydration drink is an unnatural color and packs more sugar than a can of soda, it might be time to look elsewhere for your hydration.

Determining Your Hydration Needs for Training

The first step to re-hydrating is to diagnose how much hydration you need in the first place. Since each body is different, there's no "set-in-stone" guideline for hydration or how much water you should drink. But it is important to know how to recognize the signs of dehydration.[326, 327]

- Urine color. If all is going well, your urine color should be light. Dark urine or urine so thick you can practically stand a fork in it means you're dehydrated and need more fluids immediately.

- Keep your weight up. At ultra-endurance events, they often track your body weight to see how much fluid you're losing. You want to lose pounds from fat, not from water. Keep your weight up near pre-exercise levels!

- Know the weather. Humidity, heat, and altitude are all variables you'll need to pay attention to if you want to keep properly hydrated. Be on "alert" when you exercise in these difficult conditions.

APPENDIX VIII:

Potentially Hazardous:
Water, Alcohol, and Food Additives

Water

Our simple recommendation: drink clean, filtered water—and lots of it.

H20 is the most common particle in your body, so calling it an "essential nutrient" doesn't really do it justice.

Yet, for how prevalent water is in the body, it's difficult to summarize in one sentence what it does. It helps dissolve food as soon as it hits your tongue. It helps carry nutrients to the cells. It lubricates your joints and aids in body temperature regulation. It dissolves elements into their ions, keeping your electrolytes in proper balance.

The truth is, water accomplishes so much that contributes to your health, wellness, and even your survival, that it needs its own chart:

Key Roles of Water in Human Health

Water's Role	Description
Ingredient	Water is the chief ingredient in your lungs, your kidneys, your muscles, your brain, your heart, and even represents a portion of your bones.
Medium	Without water, there is no digestion in the body and very few chemical reactions. With water as a medium, your body can execute a number of chemical reactions key to metabolism.
Regulating body temperature	We need to stay within a tight margin of 98.6 degrees Fahrenheit for good health, and water's role in both sweating and respiration allows that to happen.
Solvent	Water is an ionizing solvent, which allows your body to use elements like sodium and potassium as electrolytes. Without water playing its role in your body's electrical system, your neurons couldn't fire and your brain couldn't send command impulses to your muscles
Digestion	Water aids in digestion, acting as the first solvent your body uses—in the form of saliva—to begin breaking down food. Water is also an important tool for the kidneys to release toxins and waste from your system.
Lubrication	Joint lubrication, vital for keeping limb movement smooth and pain-free.

Immune System	Aids in maintaining moist mucus.
Energy!	Water molecules are necessary in the citric acid cycle, a metabolic process that organisms like you use to turn food into energy.
Absorption	Absorbing water-soluble vitamins, like all of the B vitamins.
Transportation	Carrying and absorbing other nutrients, including minerals, and transporting glucose.
Protection	Protecting and moistening the eyes.

See the "Danger in the water?" and Plastics sections in this Appendix for other concerns and how to make sure you're drinking not only enough, but the safest, cleanest water possible.

Alcohol

Alcohol, despite providing seven calories of energy per gram, is not truly a nutrient, thanks to the fact that it doesn't promote growth or repair once it's in your body. True, alcohol could be classified as a carbohydrate. But, unlike other carbohydrates, it can and will not be stored as glycogen in the liver. Instead, it is more readily converted to fat—fat that is often stored in the liver itself.

Like sugar, alcohol is given metabolic priority in your body. In other words, alcohol is highly toxic and has to be metabolized before any other substances you've ingested. The really bad news here is that if you hit the Taco Bell or Waffle House after drinking, your body continues to burn the beer and vodka and not the burrito and bacon. Thus the phenomenon of the beer gut.

With the liver breaking down approximately the alcohol content of four ounces of wine or one can of beer per hour, you know there's a fixed amount of alcohol that you can tolerate before intoxication—an appropriate word—begins.

There's no debate that chronically drinking too much alcohol is very, very bad for you. It directly or indirectly leads to a number of health problems, including:

• Brain damage and neural dysfunction	• Higher risk of mortality (in fact, a study published in The Lancet even found the mortality risks were not far from those of a sedentary lifestyle) [328]
• Liver disease	• Increased aging
• Weight gain	• Increased risk of some cancers, including lung and pancreatic cancers
• Cardiovascular disease	

When added to the increased risk of psychological problems caused by excessive alcohol consumption, it's apparent that drinking too much alcohol is very, very bad for you.

But you already knew that. What's less certain is how much alcohol you should consume in moderation, typically defined as one to two drinks, or enough that your liver can still break the alcohol down effectively.

Alcohol in Moderation

How much alcohol is "good" to drink? Should you abstain completely and never look back? Maybe not. A paper published as recently as 2012 noted that when compared to non-drinkers, people who consume a moderate amount of wine, daily, enjoy a number of health benefits, particularly a lower rate in mortality from cardiovascular or neurodegenerative diseases.[329] And it wasn't the only journal to find these benefits:

Alcohol in Moderation

The Benefits	Source
Moderate red wine consumption associated with "overall" improvement in health[330]	South African Medical Journal, 2005
Moderate drinking showed a health benefit to those with poor diet, little exercise, and smokers[331]	Journal of Epidemiology and Community Health, 2008
Observational studies showed alcoholic drinks were "linked" with a lower risk of heart disease[332]	British Medical Journal, 1996
Moderate alcohol consumption linked with "highest odds of reporting above-average health status"[333]	American Journal of Health Promotion, 2007

Keep in mind that alcohol isn't a nutrient, so you don't need any in your diet. If you want to abstain from alcohol completely, you might even realize similar health benefits from increased exercise or changes in your diet.

Chemicals and Food Additives

You'd be shocked to find out just how much of the "food" in your local supermarket isn't really "food" at all.

Much of the food we buy these days comes plastic-wrapped with an artificially-lengthened shelf life. Take one look at that label on your box of crackers or processed meat sticks, and you'll be amazed to find just how many chemicals, preservatives, and additives constitute the list of ingredients.

Chemicals and toxins in your food make you fat, resistant to losing weight, and are increasingly being implicated in everything from physical to emotional illness.

Chemicals and Food Additives

Flavorings, dyes, colorings, stabilizers, hydrogenated oils, preservatives, artificial sugars—it's astounding just how much of the food we eat has nothing to do with nutrition whatsoever. Some estimates suggest the average person ingests 140 to 150 pounds of additives every single year.

Remember the "Jack LaLanne" Rule

Fitness guru Jack LaLanne, who lived a healthy life all the way to the ripe old age of 96, had a rule: if God didn't make it, don't eat it!

The problem is that toxins are hard to escape. Cancer-causing chemicals are found everywhere. We usually get away with this because limited exposure to small amounts of chemicals can seem harmless—but it's not! When you're exposed to chemicals and food additives on a daily basis, the damage adds up.

The food you buy should have labels that just list real food. By avoiding foods labeled with other long words and chemical formulas you can't understand, you take a big step. Jack LaLanne, who was still pulling tugboats—with his teeth—when he was in his eighties said, "If God didn't make it, I won't eat it." That's a good rule to follow.

Here are some of the biggest offenders:

Offender	Appearance on Food Labels	Associated Health Problems	Food Sources
Artificial Colors	"Yellow (tartrazine – yellow color of boxed macaroni) No. 5," "Red No. 40," etc.	Hyperactivity in children, potential asthma aggravation[334]	Soft drinks, juices, boxed macaroni, yellow cupcakes, cheese crackers, frozen waffles
Sodium benzoate	Sodium benzoate	Increased hyperactivity in children, possible inhibition of leptin release,[335] headaches, upset stomach	Processed grain products, soft drinks, salad dressings, condiments, jams and jellies
Potassium bromate	Potassium bromate	A potential for cancer risk: in California, labels are required to come with a cancer warning if potassium bromate is present[336]	Flour and its associated products, including breads and rolls
Methylcyclopropene	Smart Fresh	A chemical sprayed on fruits to extend their shelf life, but the research is uncertain	Fruit and produce

Monosodium glutamate	Monosodium glutamate (MSG) and texturized vegetable protein (TVP)	Neurotoxins. Some people experience extreme sensitivity[337]	Packaged, canned foods

Danger in the Water?

It can take effort to find clean, fresh water. True, tap water is readily available just about anywhere in the US, from park water fountains to bathroom faucets. But once you learn what's in the water supply, you might think twice about whether or not to drink it.

- **Chlorine**. Yes, the same chemical you use to kill bacteria in your swimming pool is used in smaller amounts to accomplish the same purpose in your drinking water. The byproducts of chlorine treatment have been associated with increased cancer risk.[338]
- **Germs**. Despite the chlorine treatment, a National Resources Defense Council review found that pathogens were frequently found in municipal drinking water sources.
- **Arsenic**. Many municipal sources regularly test below the minimum safety standards, but there are those who believe that any arsenic in drinking water is unacceptable.
- **Lead**. Like it or not, many cities rely on old pumps to move their water, and problems with these pumps can result in trace amounts of lead getting into the supplies. The NRDC's tests found lead was a frequent offender across different water sources.

Plastics

Plastics are so prevalent in our foods that the government has even established an average daily amount we can safely ingest.

What don't we consume that has already been in plastic? Even plastic water bottles and broccoli heated in plastic ware can expose us to high levels of phthalates, a substance added to make plastic more flexible.

BPA-Free?

Although it's good to find bottles that are BPA-free, if it's plastic, it still contains phthalates.

Needless to say, plastics are not meant to be in your body. They're associated with a number of health problems, including:

Decreased sex drive
Damaged hormone receptors
Fatigue
Prostate, breast, lung, and thyroid cancers

Another problem is that many plastics contain bisphenol A, or BPA. This substance is so controversial that it is even illegal in some countries, and has shown a number of negative health effects eerily similar to those listed above.

Filtering your water and drinking out of glass or stainless steel glasses and bottles are yet two other important keys to well being.

Toxins—To Go!

Other problems to be aware of are polystyrene present in your to-go Styrofoam cups and containers. It's easier for these substances to get into your foods and fluids when they're heated, which is an important fact to keep in mind when pouring yourself hot coffee in a Styrofoam cup.

In order to avoid plastics, it's best to keep cooking at home, where you're free to choose your own containers, bottles, and serving dishes. The more you rely on prepackaged and processed foods, the more likely you'll be exposed to plastics.

Styrofoam cups, plates, and food holders contain this polystyrene, which get into foods especially when they've been heated.

Heavy Metals

Heavy metals are scary, because they can act as neurotoxins, or nerve and brain poisons. People are rightly cautious about small amounts of mercury in their fish. But there are other potential heavy metals that you'll want to be aware of as well:

Heavy Metals	Products and Foods to Avoid
Aluminum	Personal hygiene products heavy in aluminum, household appliances.
Cadmium	Foods contaminated by cadmium-rich fertilizers, typically farm crops.
Mercury	The NRDC recommends avoiding swordfish, shark, marlin, mackerel, orange roughy, tilefish, and tuna (bigeye, and ahi).[339] Also in amalgam fillings.
Lead	Poor municipal water sources, lead-based paint in older house.[340]
Antimony	Often found in the soil, which represents a threat to water supplies, as well as foods that grow in contaminated soils.
Arsenic	Found in the water supply or in soils.

As the above chart demonstrates, reducing your exposure to heavy metals will rely on getting your plants and water from clean sources that are free of contaminants. In the case of mercury, you can avoid the fish listed and enjoy other seafood like herring, wild salmon, and sardines.

How to Avoid Contaminants
in Your Produce

When you consider just how many commercial farmers have allowed contaminants like antimony into their fertilizers, their soil, and ultimately their food, you begin to realize the importance of getting whole, naturally-grown foods.

Just as it's important to get grass-fed and pasture-raised sources for your meats, dairy, and eggs, it's also important to get your vegetables from the highest-quality sources if you want to avoid contaminants. Farmer's markets are good ways to find out about the source of your food as well as discover local organic farmers and the quality of their soil.

Sadly, chemicals are too prevalent today to allow any one individual totally avoid chemicals and contaminants. But you can do your best to be conscious of which produce typically is highest in pesticides and inorganic chemicals so you can be sure that you buy them organic.

The Environmental Working Group puts out a "Dirty Dozen" list each year. Go to www. ewg.org for annual updates. By choosing these and other produce as organic you can reduce your chemical exposure by up to ninety percent. Organic foods also have higher nutrient values.[341, 342]

These are the most recent "Dirty Dozen" list of produce items you should buy organic:

- Apples
- Strawberries
- Grapes
- Celery
- Peaches
- Spinach
- Sweet bell peppers
- Nectarines
- Cucumbers
- Potatoes
- Cherry Tomatoes
- Hot Peppers

It's not always necessary that you spend top-dollar to get food that is low in contaminants and healthy for you. What's really required is that you spend your grocery money consciously, knowing which foods truly represent the best possible nutrients and the fewest contaminants.

APPENDIX IX:

Soaking and Sprouting
Making Nuts, Grains, Seeds, and Beans More Edible

Nuts, grains, beans, and seeds are designed to stay alive and intact until time to sprout and grow. As a result, nature has placed within them an internal defense system that causes these foods to be anti-nutrients or even toxic in high doses. These things have become a common part of our diets, but contain substances that can inhibit your food-digesting enzymes and that can block the absorption of key minerals.

If you think of proper growing conditions, these seed-based foods become wet over time so they can germinate and reproduce themselves as the plant foods we eat. In a nutshell, pun-intended, this is why we need to soak and sprout these nutrients to make them safer to eat. As they go through the soaking and sprouting process, the substances that create problems in human health can be reduced or eliminated.

Soaking nuts, beans, and seeds, and sprouting grains, also serves to increase the presences of vitamins, particularly B vitamins, reduce the presences of unhealthy tannins, enhance the production of digestive enzymes, break down unhealthy gluten, and provide several other benefits.

Below are the basics to soaking and sprouting. Other options can be easily found on-line. It's a popular topic. Given the challenges related to these foods, these should be eaten in moderation.

Some Basic Nut, Seed, and Bean Soaking Instructions
1. Use water with approximately 1 Tbsp of salt. Some methods recommend adding an acidic agent, like lemon juice. Beans can also be soaked in vinegar.
2. Minimum time to see results is seven hours with best results coming in twelve to twenty-four hours.
3. Eat nuts and seeds wet or dry in a dehydrator

Basic Sprouting Instructions
How to Sprout Grain:
1. Rinse the grains
2. Place them in a glass or stainless steel container and fill with warm water until the water is two to three inches above the grain
3. Soak the grains for twelve hours/overnight
4. After the time is up, pour out the water through a screen filter a mesh cloth and leave them moist in the container.
5. Rinse the grains multiple times, stirring so you get all of them evenly
6. Rinse the grains occasionally over the course of one to three days until you see the buds appearing as they begin to sprout
7. Drain them, refrigerate, or use a dehydrator if you're going to grind for use as flour.

APPENDIX X:

Shopping List

*Organic where possible is ideal

Produce:

• Arugula	• Kale
• Avocado	• Onion (red, white)
• Brussels sprouts	• Broccoli
• Cabbage	• Cilantro
• Cauliflower	• Ginger
• Celery	• Garlic
• Snow Peas	• Jicama
• Cucumber	• Berries of your choice (fresh or frozen)
• Greens for salad (romaine, spinach, mixed greens, etc.)	• Green apples
• Scallions or green onions	• Bell peppers (red, green, yellow)
• Green beans	• Mint leaves
• Organic tomatoes (regular or cherry)	• Tarragon leaves
• Zucchini	• Sage leaves
• Mushrooms	• Fresh dill

Milk and Dairy:

• Coconut milk	• Sour cream
• Organic or fee-range eggs	• Heavy cream
• Whole Greek or goat milk yogurt	• Brie cheese
• Raw or organic unsalted butter	• Mozzarella cheese
• Organic cream cheese	• Organic cheddar cheese
• Organic cottage cheese	• Organic Monterey Jack cheese

Meat, Poultry, Wild-Caught Fish:

• Organic or grass-fed beef or bison (steak, ground)

- Organic or grass-fed chicken (breast, wings, and quarters)
- Organic or grass-fed turkey (breast, ground)
- Salmon and smoked, canned salmon
- Tilapia
- Sardines (canned)

Spices:

• Celtic sea salt	• Coriander
• Ground cinnamon	• Turmeric
• Ground nutmeg	• Chili powder
• Black pepper or peppercorns	• Basil leaves
• Garlic powder	• Ground ginger

Miscellaneous:

- Maximized Living Perfect Protein, Vanilla and Chocolate
- Red wine
- Lemon or lime Juice
- Dry white wine

Baking Aisle:

• Coconut flour	• Xylitol
• Blanched almond flour	• Pure vanilla extract
• Golden flax meal	• Lemon zest
• Organic rolled oats or gluten-free	• Baking soda
• Coconut oil—extra virgin	• Unsweetened coconut (shredded or flakes)
• Sesame oil	• Unsweetened or organic baking chocolate 73%> (square, chips)
• Olive oil	• Cocoa powder
• Stevia	

Condiments:

• Apple cider	• Hot sauce
• vinegar	• White vinegar
• Balsamic vinegar	• Tomato paste
• Almond or peanut	• Tomato sauce
• butter	• Organic salsa
• Bragg's Liquid Amino	• Mustard
• Organic tamari	• Black olives
• Dijon mustard	

Nuts and Seeds:

- Raw or organic almonds, pecans, walnuts, hazelnuts
- Chia seeds
- Flax seeds

Recipe Index with Nutrient Analysis

*Organic where possible is ideal

Berry Smoothie

Ingredients:
1 cup of berries (strawberries, blueberries, blackberries, raspberries, or combination)
1/2 cup coconut milk
Water and 1–2 cups of crushed ice, depending on desired thickness, consistency
1 scoop Vanilla Perfect Protein
1/4 cup of flax and/or chia seeds

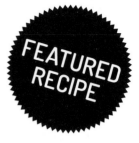

Directions:
Blend together until you've achieved the desired consistency

Breadless Bread

Ingredients:
2 tablespoons coconut flour
2 cups blanched almond flour
1/4 cup golden flax meal
1/4 teaspoon Celtic sea salt
1/2 teaspoon baking soda
5 eggs
1 Tbsp coconut oil
1 Tbsp xylitol
1 tablespoon apple cider vinegar

Directions:
Place almond flour, coconut flour, flax, salt and baking soda in a food processor.
Pulse ingredients together. Pulse in eggs, oil, xylitol, and vinegar. Pour batter into a greased 7.5 x 3.5 Magic Line loaf pan. Bake at 350° for 30 minutes. Cool and serve.

Blueberry Muffins (ten muffins)

Ingredients:
3 organic eggs
1/2 cup whole milk Greek yogurt
1/3 cup grape-seed oil
1/2 cup xylitol
1 Tbsp vanilla extract
1/2 cup coconut flour
1/4 tsp sea salt
1/4 tsp baking soda
1 cup fresh or frozen blueberries

Directions:
Preheat oven to 350 and line muffin tins. In a food processor combine eggs, yogurt, oil, vanilla and xylitol. Pulse until mixed. Pulse in coconut flour, salt and baking soda. Add blueberries and pulse two or three times to break up slightly. Fill lined muffin tins. Bake for 20–25 minutes until tops are slightly browned. Makes 10 muffins.

Nutrition data per muffin:
145 kcals
10 grams fat, 5 grams monounsaturated, 3 grams saturated, 2 grams polyunsaturated)
9 grams carbohydrate
4 grams fiber
5 grams protein

Brownies
(Serves 16. Serving Size: 1 brownie)

Ingredients:
1 stick butter (raw or organic)
3 oz unsweetened, organic baking chocolate (3 squares) or unsweetened cocoa powder
1 1/2 cup 100% Egg Protein (Vitol)
 Stevia to taste
1 Tbsp pure vanilla extract
3 eggs (free-range)
2/3 cup flax seed ground or flax meal
1/2 tsp baking soda

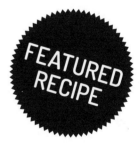

Directions:
Preheat oven to 325°. Lightly grease a 9x9 baking pan. Melt butter and chocolate in a small saucepan on low heat. Stir until smooth and allow to cool. Add Vitol, stevia, vanilla, and eggs and beat well. Combine flax seeds, baking soda, and add to the chocolate mixture. Add chopped walnuts if using.

Spread mixture into baking pan and bake for 25 minutes at 325°. When done, remove and cool brownies in pan on a wire rack. When cool, slice and serve.
Note: *For moister brownies, reduce cooking time to 20 minutes. For a smoother texture soak flax seeds for 20–30 minutes in just enough water to cover them. Drain any excess before using in recipe.*

Brownie Cereal

Ingredients:
1 1/2 cups unsweetened shredded coconut
1/3 cup unsweetened coconut milk
1/4 cup unsweetened cocoa powder
1/2 teaspoon liquid or powder stevia to taste
1/2 teaspoon vanilla extract

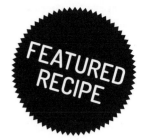

Directions:
Preheat oven to 350F. Blend in a stainless steel pot at medium heat the coconut milk and cocoa powder. Add in the stevia and coconut until it's all blended in and remove from heat. Spread mixture into a thin layer on a parchment on a baking sheet. Bake at 350F for 25–30 minutes dependent on how crunchy you like it. Stir the cereal about 15 minutes and make sure it doesn't burn. Store in airtight container.

Cauliflower Crust Veggie Pizza

Ingredients:
2 cups cauliflower florets
1/2 cup shredded mozzarella cheese
1 egg
1 Tbsp olive oil
1/2 cup tomato sauce mixed with 1/2 tsp Italian seasoning, 1/2 tsp minced garlic, and 1/2 tsp sea salt
1/2 cup mushrooms
1/2 cup sliced olives

Directions:
Preheat oven to 425 degrees. Grease cookie sheet with butter or coconut oil. Grate the cauliflower with a cheese grater. Place in water in a stainless steel pan and cook for 12 minutes. Mix together the grated cauliflower, egg, and half of the cheese. Transfer to the cookie sheet, and using your hands, pat out into a round about 1/4" thick. Brush olive oil over top of crust. Bake for 15 minutes. Remove from oven. Add tomato sauce, remaining cheese, mushrooms, and olives. Return to oven for 5–10 minutes, just until cheese is melted.

Chia Seed Cocoa Almond Pudding
(1 serving)
Ingredients:
1 Tbsp chia seeds
1 Tbsp almond butter
1 tsp cocoa powder
1/2 tsp cinnamon
1/2 tsp sea salt
Stevia or xylitol to taste

Directions:
Mix chia seeds with 1/2 cup water and let soak at least four hours. Stir in remaining ingredients.

Nutrition data per serving:
185 kcals
13 grams fat (7 grams monounsaturated, 1 gram saturated, 5 grams polyunsaturated)
10 grams carbohydrate
6 grams fiber
6 grams protein

Chicken Wings
(4 servings)
Ingredients:
1/4 cup unsalted butter (ideally raw, grass-fed)
1 teaspoon granulated stevia
1/4 cup red wine (optional)
1/4 cup liquid aminos or organic tamari
2 Tbsp fresh lemon juice
1 teaspoons Dijon mustard
1/8 cup hot sauce (adjust to your taste)
2 pounds organic chicken wings
1 teaspoons sea salt
1/8 teaspoon black pepper
1 teaspoons garlic powder

Directions:
Preheat oven to 350° F. Melt butter in a small–medium saucepan over medium heat. Add the stevia, wine, tamari, lemon juice, Dijon mustard, hot sauce, salt, pepper, and garlic powder and mix. In a large bowl, mix the chicken wings with the sauce. Arrange chicken wings on a large baking sheet lined with parchment paper. Bake wings at 350° F for 35–40 minutes or until chicken is done. For even more tender wings with a further reduced sauce, reduce heat to 250° F and continue cooking for 3–4 hours, flipping about every 30 minutes.

Nutrition data per serving:
335 kcals
27 grams fat (10 grams monounsaturated, 13 grams saturated, 4 grams polyunsaturated)
1 gram carbohydrate
0 gram fiber
22 grams protein

Chinese Chicken Salad
(2 servings)

Ingredients:
12 oz skinless cooked organic chicken breast, cut into thin strips
4 cups shredded cabbage
3 cups diced jicama
1 cup minced celery
4 sliced scallions
1/4 cup chopped peanuts
2 tsp cilantro
1 tsp ginger
1/2 tsp minced garlic
2 tsp low-sodium soy sauce
2 tsp lime juice
2 Tbsp sesame oil
2 Tbsp olive oil

Directions:
In food processor blend ginger, garlic, soy sauce, lime juice, sesame and olive oil.
Combine dressing with chicken, cabbage, jicama, celery, and scallions, in a large bowl.
Place chicken salad on plates and sprinkle with peanuts and cilantro.

Nutrition data per serving:
645 kcals
42 grams fat (19 grams monounsaturated, 8 grams saturated, 15 grams polyunsaturated)
26 grams carbohydrate
13 grams fiber
40 grams protein

Chocolate Almond Butter Fudge
(8 servings)
Ingredients:
1 cup dark chocolate chips (73% dark)
1 cup almond butter
2 tbsp xylitol
1/2 tbsp vanilla extract
1/4 tsp sea salt

Directions:
Melt chocolate in medium pot. Remove from heat and stir in almond butter and xylitol. Once incorporated, stir in vanilla and salt. Spread into a loaf pan and refrigerate for at least 2 hours. Cut quickly into small squares and store in fridge or freezer.
Note: if using unsweetened chocolate, use more xylitol. If chocolate is less than 73% dark, eliminate xylitol.

Nutrition data per serving:
350 kcals
28 grams fat (16 grams monounsaturated, 7 grams saturated, 5 grams polyunsaturated)
18 grams carbohydrate
5 grams fiber
6 grams protein

Chocolate Avocado Pudding
(1 serving)
Ingredients:
1 avocado, soft and ripe
1 teaspoon vanilla
1/4 cup cocoa powder
stevia to taste
6 tablespoons coconut milk
1/4 cup of ice
(Even better with a scoop of Perfect Protein)

Directions:
Cut avocado in half and remove pit. Scoop out flesh and put it in the blender along with remaining ingredients. Process until smooth, occasionally scraping down sides. Serve immediately or refrigerate until ready to serve. Ice keeps it from getting hot in the blender so you can eat it right away.

Nutrition data per serving:
580 kcals
47 grams fat (18 grams monounsaturated, 25 grams saturated, 4 grams polyunsaturated)
29 grams carbohydrate
16 grams fiber
10 grams protein

Chocolate Covered Strawberry Smoothie

Ingredients:

1 cup coconut milk

1–2 cups of ice depending on desired thickness, consistency

1/2 avocado (makes it like a malted)

1 1/2 cups of strawberries

2–3 tablespoons of unsweetened cocoa powder

1 scoop Chocolate Perfect Protein

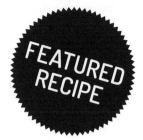

Directions:

Mix ingredients in a blender until desired consistency

Chocolate Malted Smoothie

Ingredients:

1 cup coconut milk

1–2 cups of ice depending on desired thickness, consistency

1/2 avocado (Makes it like a malted)

1 tablespoon of almond or peanut butter

2–3 tablespoons of unsweetened cocoa powder

1 scoop Chocolate Perfect Protein

Directions:

Mix ingredients in a blender until desired consistency.

Cinnamon Almonds

(8 servings)

Ingredients:

1 egg white

1 Tbsp vanilla extract

2 cups raw almonds

2/3 cup stevia or xylitol

1 teaspoon salt

1/2 teaspoon ground cinnamon

Directions:

In a large bowl, beat egg white until frothy; beat in vanilla. Add almonds; stir gently to coat. Combine the sugar substitute, salt and cinnamon; add to nut mixture and stir gently to coat. Spread evenly into a greased 15-in. x 10-in. x 1-in. baking pan. Bake at 300° for 25–30 minutes or until almonds are crisp, stirring once. Cool. Store in an airtight container.

Nutrition data per serving:

215 kcals

17 grams fat (12 grams monounsaturated, 1 gram saturated, 4 grams polyunsaturated)

7 grams carbohydrate

4 grams fiber

9 grams protein

Cinnamon Pancakes
(serves 2)

Ingredients:

1 Tbsp coconut oil

2 eggs

6 Tbsp water

1/4 tsp salt

4 Tbsp almond flour

2 scoops Maximized Living Vanilla Protein Powder

1 tsp vanilla extract

stevia or xylitol to taste

2 tsp butter (ideally raw, grass-fed)

Toppings:

1 1/2 Tbsp butter

2 tsp cinnamon and stevia or xylitol to taste

Directions:

Melt coconut oil in small stainless steel pan. Add eggs and whisk together. Add water, salt, vanilla extract, almond flour, whey protein powder and stevia or xylitol, beating well after each addition. Melt butter in medium-sized skillet over low heat. Pour 1/2 of batter into pan. Once edges have set and begun to turn light golden brown, flip over with a spatula. Cook on the other side for 1–2 minutes. Transfer to plate. Repeat with remaining batter. Mix cinnamon and stevia or xylitol in small bowl. Top each pancake with butter and cinnamon mixture.

Nutrition data per serving:

450 kcals

29 grams fat (10 grams monounsaturated, 17 grams saturated, 2 grams polyunsaturated)

19 grams carbohydrate

11 grams fiber

28 grams protein

Coconut Macaroons
(12 macaroons)

Ingredients:

1 cup organic raw almonds

2 cups unsweetened coconut flakes

1 scoop Maximized Living Vanilla Protein Powder

3 Tbsp organic unsweetened cocoa

stevia or xylitol to taste.

7 Tbsp warm (liquid) coconut oil

1 Tbsp flax seeds

Directions:

In blender or food processor grind almonds, and flax seeds. Blend in remaining ingredients. Remove mixture and place tablespoon-sized macaroons on a cookie sheet or shallow baking dish and chill.

Nutrition data per macaroon:
200 kcals
17 grams fat (5 grams monounsaturated, 8 grams saturated, 2 grams polyunsaturated)
6 grams carbohydrate
3 grams fiber
5 grams protein

Eggnog smoothie
(serves 1)

Ingredients:
1 scoop of Whey protein powder
1/2 can coconut milk (full-fat)
1/2 avocado
1–2 cups ice to desired thickness and consistency
2 capfuls vanilla extract
2 tsp ground nutmeg, plus cinnamon and stevia to taste

Directions:
Into blender container add all ingredients. Blend on high until creamy and frothy. Serve immediately.

Grainless Granola
(2 servings)

Ingredients:
1/4 cup whole organic flax seeds
1/4 cup raw organic almonds
1/4 cup dry, unsweetened coconut
2 tsp dried mint leaves or 2 mint tea bags
1/2 cup coconut milk (for use as Cereal)

Directions:
In blender or food processor, pour flax seeds, almonds, and dry coconut through opening in top of cover. Replace removable cap and continue processing until ingredients are reduced to a chunky, grain-like consistency, about 1 minute. Stop motor, scrape down to loosen mixture in bottom of blender or bowl, if necessary. Add loose, dry mint leaves or open 2 mint tea bags and dump contents. Process a few more bursts until blended. Pour 1/4 cup coconut milk over each serving of cereal and enjoy.

Can be enjoyed cold or let stand a few minutes and warm slightly on stove top for a "hot" cereal experience. Flax seeds will thicken mixture as it sits.

Nutrition data per serving:
265 kcals
20 grams fat (6 grams monounsaturated, 10 grams saturated, 5 grams polyunsaturated)
12 grams carbohydrate
8 grams fiber
9 grams protein

Lemon Cheesecake

Crust Ingredients:
3/4 c pecans
2 tsp xylitol
3/4 cup almonds
4 Tbsp melted butter

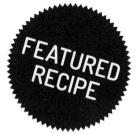

Directions for crust:
Mix the dry ingredients in a bowl. Add melted butter & stir until well mixed. Pour mixture into spring form pan, shake, spread around, and pat down firmly. Bake at 350 for 10 minutes or until starting to brown. Cool crust, then wrap pan in foil to prepare for baking the filling.

Filling Ingredients:
1 1/2 lb cream cheese at room temp
3 large eggs at room temp
1 cup sour cream
2 tsp lemon zest
2 cup xylitol
2 Tbsp fresh lemon juice

Directions for filling:
In large bowl beat cream cheese until smooth then add sour cream and beat until fluffy. Gradually add xylitol. Beat in eggs one at a time until fully incorporated. Mix in lemon zest and lemon juice. Pour mixture over cooled crust, place in pan, and fill pan around pan half-way with boiling water. Bake at 325 for 60–75 min. until center is almost set but still slightly jiggly. Allow to cool.

Lemon Curd (Topping for cheesecake)

Ingredients:
1 1/2 tsp lemon zest
1 egg at room temp
6 Tbsp fresh lemon juice
1 egg yolk
1/2 xylitol
2 Tbsp unsalted butter, cut into bits

Directions:
Make in top of double boiler. Combine lemon zest, lemon juice, egg, egg yolk and xylitol. Gently heat. Whisk until hot and frothy, about 5 min. Gradually whisk in butter and continue whisking for 7 min. or until thickened and coats back of spoon. Remove from heat and let cool for 30 min.

Remove cheesecake from pan by running thin blade around the edge of pan. Remove side and transfer to serving plate. Spread lemon curd on top. Cool in frig for 2 hrs or overnight before cutting.

Pepper Steak

(4 servings)

Ingredients:

1 lb grass-fed beef or bison rib eye steaks

2-3 Tbsp dried green and black peppercorns

1 tsp sea salt

1 tsp grated lemon zest

1 med garlic clove, smashed

1 tsp tamari

Directions:

Crush peppercorns with back of spoon or in grinder. Mix with sea salt, garlic, tamari, and lemon zest. Press mixture all over steaks. Let marinate with this coating for at least a few minutes. Sear steaks by broiling in oven broiler, over the grill, or in heavy cast iron skillet on medium high heat, 3 minutes on a side.

Nutrition data per serving:

240 kcals

21 grams protein

17 grams fat (8 grams monounsaturated, 7 grams saturated, 2 grams polyunsaturated)

Protein Almond Bars

Ingredients:

2 cups raw almonds

1/2 cup flax seed meal

1/2 cup unsweetened shredded coconut

2 scoops of Organic Whey Protein, flavor of your choice

1/2 cup raw almond butter

1/2 teaspoon sea salt

1/2 cup coconut oil

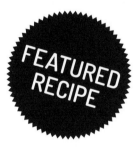

1/4 tsp. of KAL brand stevia, or equivalent, to taste (This is the sweetening power equivalent of approximately 1/2 cup of sugar). Taste, and adjust to your liking.

1 tablespoon pure vanilla extract (No sugar—check the label)

8 squares unsweetened chocolate, melted and sweetened to taste with stevia and cinnamon (optional)

Directions:

Place almonds, flax meal, shredded coconut, Organic Whey Protein, almond butter and salt in a food processor. Pulse briefly, about 10 seconds. In a small sauce pan, melt coconut oil over very low heat. Remove coconut oil from stove; stir stevia and vanilla into oil. Add coconut oil mixture to food processor and pulse until ingredients form a coarse paste. Press mixture into an 8 x 8 glass baking dish. (A parchment paper liner helps when you want to remove the bars from the dish.) Chill in refrigerator for 1 hour, until mixture hardens.

In a double boiler, melt chocolate, stirring in stevia and cinnamon.
Spread melted chocolate over bars; return to refrigerator for 30 minutes, until chocolate hardens. Remove from refrigerator, cut into bars, and serve.

Roast Chicken and Cauli-rice
(6 servings)

Ingredients:
Whole organic chicken (about 4 lbs)
1 tsp sea salt
1 tsp pepper
1 tsp garlic powder
1 tbsp grape-seed oil

Cauliflower Rice
1 large head cauliflower, chopped
1 small onion, diced
1 celery stalk, diced
2 Tbsp coconut oil
Sea salt and pepper to taste

Directions:
Preheat oven to 375 degrees. Prepare chicken by rinsing and patting dry. Place whole chicken, breast up, in an 11x7 baking pan or a roasting pan. Rub chicken with oil and sprinkle seasonings evenly over the top. Cover with foil and bake for about 1 hour. Remove foil and bake an additional 30-45 minutes until thickest part of breast reaches 160 degrees and skin browns.

Place cauliflower in food processor and pulse until it is the consistency of rice grains. In a large skillet heat oil over med/high heat. Add onion and celery and cook until soft. Add cauliflower to pan and continue to cook for about 20 minutes, stirring occasionally until cauli-rice just starts to brown. Season with salt and pepper to taste.

Nutrition data per serving:
405 kcals
23 grams fat (12 grams monounsaturated, 6 grams saturated, 5 grams polyunsaturated)
11 grams carbohydrate
4 grams fiber
39 grams protein

Salmon with Basil Cream Sauce
(4 servings)

Ingredients:

For salmon:
4 salmon steaks (6 oz each)
1/4 cup olive oil
1 Tbsp lemon juice
Sea salt and fresh ground black pepper to taste

For sauce:
20 fresh basil leaves
1/3 cup dry white wine
2 cloves garlic
1 cup heavy cream
1 Tbsp fresh lemon juice
2 Tbsp unsalted raw grass-fed butter
Sea salt and fresh ground black pepper to taste

Directions:
Preheat grill to high. Rinse salmon under cold water, drain, and blot dry. Brush salmon on both sides with olive oil. Season with lemon juice, salt and pepper. Combine basil, wine, and garlic in a blender and process until a smooth puree forms. Transfer to a small heavy saucepan. Stir in cream. Bring to a simmer over medium heat, taking care not to let cream boil over. Stir frequently for 10–15 minutes, until sauce is reduced by half. Add butter and lemon juice, continuing to stir. Once the butter is incorporated into the cream mixture, remove from heat and season with salt and pepper. Cover and keep warm. Grill salmon until it just starts to fully flake. Remove from heat. Spoon sauce over salmon and serve.

Nutrition data per serving:
550 kcals
45 grams fat (20 grams monounsaturated, 20 grams saturated, 5 grams polyunsaturated)
2 grams carbohydrate
0 grams fiber
35 grams protein

Chicken Curry
(4 servings)

Ingredients:
1/4 cup coconut oil
1 cup chopped onion
2 tsp sea salt
2 tsp chopped garlic
2 tsp ground ginger
2 tsp coriander
1 tsp turmeric
1 tsp chili powder
4 cups broccoli florets
2 cups snow peas
2 cups mushrooms
1/2 cup coconut milk
1 lb chicken breast, diced

Directions:
Heat oil in a wok or large saucepan over medium-high heat. Add the onion, then cook and stir until browned. Mix in garlic and spices. Add broccoli, pea pods, and mushrooms. Cook and stir for 1–2 minutes. Add coconut milk and chicken. Continue cooking for 10–12 minutes, until chicken is no longer pink. Stir and remove from heat.

Nutrition data per serving:
445 kcals
23 grams fat (4 grams monounsaturated, 17 grams saturated, 2 grams polyunsaturated)
21 grams carbohydrate
6 grams fiber
38 grams protein

Green Smoothie

Ingredients:
2 cups of kale, 1 head romaine lettuce, 2 cups spinach, or combo of the 3
1/2 cup coconut milk
1 scoop Vanilla or Chocolate Perfect Protein
2–3 tablespoons cocoa powder
1/2 avocado
1–2 cups of crushed ice depending on desired consistency
Stevia to taste

Directions:
Put the lettuce, kale, and/or spinach in the blender with avocado and the coconut milk. Blend until greens are fully mixed. Add ice, cocoa powder, and Perfect Protein and mix until well blended.

"Kitchen Sink" Yogurt

Ingredients:
Organic plain whole or goat's milk yogurt—if your are
dairy sensitive
Shaved unsweetened chocolate
Stevia to taste
1 cup raspberries, blueberries, strawberries, or combo
1/4 cup ground flax seed and/or chia seeds
Optional:
Shredded coconut
1 tsp almond or peanut butter
Directions: Mix together in bowl.

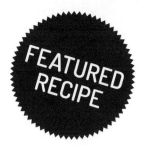

Mixed Sweet Nut Recipe

Ingredients:
5 cups of raw, whole almonds and/or pecans
1 Egg white
Tbsp of water
1/2 cup xylitol
1 Tbsp cinnamon
Pinch of salt

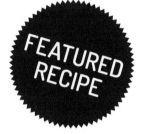

Directions:
Beat the entire mixture together. Cook for 15 min. at 350 degrees. Stir and cook for
another 10–15 min. until browned.

No-Guilt Chocolate Chip Cookies
(see? It's not all hopeless!)

Ingredients:
2 1/2 cups almond flour
1/4 teaspoon sea salt
1/4 teaspoon baking soda
1/2–3/4 cup xylitol or if using stevia, add to taste.
1 organic egg
1 tablespoon vanilla
1 stick (8 tablespoons) organic butter
1 bar sugarless chocolate, chopped into chunks.

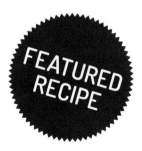

Directions:
Preheat oven to 350 degrees. Combine all the dry ingredients in a medium sized bowl. Melt
the butter gently in a saucepan. In a separate bowl, mix the butter with the egg and vanilla.
Add the wet ingredients to the dry ingredients and mix well. Chop the chocolate bar and
mix into the batter. Drop about a tablespoon of batter an inch apart on a baking sheet. Bake
until slightly brown around the edges.

Strawberry Smoothie
(1 serving)

Ingredients:
1 scoop Maximized Living Vanilla Protein Powder
1 cup frozen strawberries
1/4 cup whole milk Greek yogurt
1/2 cup coconut milk
1/4 cup flax seeds

Directions:
Place all ingredients in blender and blend until smooth.

Nutrition data per serving:
315 kcals
12 grams fat (8 grams monounsaturated, 2 grams saturated, 2 grams polyunsaturated)
24 grams carbohydrate
8 grams fiber
28 grams protein

Stuffed Pepper
(2 servings)

Ingredients:
2 large red bell peppers
10 oz ground grass-fed beef (ideally) or organic lean turkey
1/2 cup chopped onion
1/2 tsp chopped garlic
1/2 cup tomato paste
1 tsp sea salt
1 tsp mustard
2 tsp chili powder

Directions:
Preheat oven to 350 degrees. Rinse bell pepper, cut off top and remove stems and seeds from inside. Lightly grease a baking sheet with butter or coconut oil. Bake 35 minutes on middle rack. In a large non-stick skillet, over medium-high heat, add ground turkey, onion, and garlic. Cook about 10 minutes or until no longer pink. To turkey mixture, add, tomato paste, sea salt, mustard, and chili powder. Mix until all ingredients are well incorporated. Reduce heat to low and simmer 5–10 minutes. Stuff peppers with turkey mixture and serve immediately.

Nutrition data per serving:
400 kcals
17 grams fat (7 grams monounsaturated, 5 gram saturated, 5 grams polyunsaturated)
20 grams carbohydrate
6 grams fiber
41 grams protein

Turkey Burgers
(4 servings)

Ingredients:
1 lb organic lean ground turkey
1/2 cup finely chopped zucchini
1/4 cup chopped red onion
1 Tbsp fresh or dried tarragon leaves
1 Tbsp Dijon mustard
1/2 tsp sea salt
1/2 tsp pepper
2 eggs

Directions:
Preheat broiler. In mixing bowl, combine ground turkey with zucchini, onion, tarragon, mustard, salt, pepper, and eggs. Mix thoroughly. Shape into patties. Place on broiler pan. Broil 5 minutes on a side until browned. Serve immediately.

Nutrition data per serving:
275 kcals
20 grams fat (13 grams monounsaturated, 6 grams saturated, 1 gram polyunsaturated)
1 gram carbohydrate
0.5 gram fiber
23 grams protein

Turkey Meatloaf
(4 servings)

Ingredients:
1 lb organic lean ground turkey
1 organic egg
1 cup tomato sauce
1 tsp sea salt
1 tsp black pepper
1/2 cup chopped sweet onion
1/4 cup chopped organic bell pepper
1/2 cup organic rolled oats
1 tsp fresh chopped basil leaves
1 crushed garlic clove

Directions:
Preheat oven to 350 degrees. Beat egg in large mixing bowl. Add remaining ingredients except for 1/2 cup of tomato sauce and mix well. Place in glass oven baking dish and pour 1/2 cup tomato sauce on top and bake for 45–50 minutes.

Nutrition data per serving:
220 kcals
10 grams fat (6 grams monounsaturated, 2 grams saturated, 2 grams polyunsaturated)
13 grams carbohydrate
1 gram fiber
19 grams protein

Warm Steak Salad with Mushroom Brown Butter
(2 servings)

Ingredients:

12 oz grass-fed steak

2 cups mushrooms

10 fresh sage leaves

4 cups spinach

4 Tbsp butter (ideally raw, grass-fed)Salt and pepper to taste

Directions:

Sprinkle steak with salt and pepper. Broil until medium or medium-rare. Slice steak thinly across the grain. In a large skillet over medium heat, melt butter and cook until just beginning to brown, about 3 to 4 minutes. Add mushrooms and sage and sauté about 4 minutes more. Arrange spinach leaves on large plate and place sliced steak on top. Pour mushroom sauce over each and sprinkle with salt and pepper, if desired. Serve immediately.

Nutrition data per serving:

520 kcals

38 grams fat (16 grams monounsaturated, 20 grams saturated, 2 grams polyunsaturated)

5 grams carbohydrate

3 grams fiber

40 grams protein

Yogurt vegetable dip

Ingredients:

2 cups plain Greek or goat's milk yogurt

1 cup diced cucumber

2 tbsp finely chopped fresh dill

2 tbsp fresh lemon juice

2 cloves of minced garlic

Salt and pepper to taste

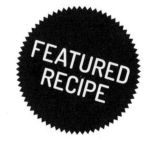

Directions:

Combine yogurt, cucumber, garlic, lemon juice, and dill. Add salt and pepper to taste. Chill before serving.

BIBLIOGRAPHY

Citations

1. WE., Lands. Diets could prevent many diseases. Lipids. 2003.
2. Mann T, Tomiyama AJ, Westling E, Lew AM, Samuels B, Chatman J. Medicare's search for effective obesity treatments: diets are not the answer. Am Psychol. Apr 2007, pp. 220-33.
3. Phys.org. [Online] http://phys.org/news94906931.html#jCp.
4. Flegal KM, Carroll MD, Ogden CL, Curtin LR. Prevalence and trends in obesity among US adults, 1999-2008. JAMA. . Jan 20, 2010 , pp. 235-41.
5. Freedman DS, Zuguo M, Srinivasan SR, Berenson GS, Dietz WH. Cardiovascular risk factors and excess adiposity among overweight children and adolescents: the Bogalusa Heart Study. Journal of Pediatrics. 2007, pp. 12–17.
6. Statistical Fact Sheet--2013 Update. s.l. : American Heart Association.
7. CDC.gov. [Online] http://www.cdc.gov/obesity/data/adult.html.
8. Putnam, J., Allshouse, J., Kantor, LS. U.S. Per Capita Food Supply Trends: More Calories, Refined Carbohydrates, and Fats. FoodReview. 2002.
9. Heart Disease and Stroke Statistics—2013 Update. Circulation. 2013.
10. Lands, B. A critique of paradoxes in current advice on dietary lipids. Prog Lipid Res. 2008.
11. PubMed Health. Metabolic Syndrome. [Online] http://www.ncbi.nlm.nih.gov/pubmedhealth/PMH0004546/
12. Krauss, et. al. Change in dietary saturated fat intake is correlated with change in mass of large low-density-lipoprotein particles in men. Am J Clin Nutr. 1998.
13. Friedman, et al. "Leptin and the regulation of body weight in mammals." Nature. 1998
14. Bowers, et. al. Ghrelin, appetite, and gastric motility: the emerging role of the stomach as an endocrine organ. The FASEB Journal. 2004.
15. Pedrosa C, Oliveira BM, Albuquerque I, Simões-Pereira C, Vaz-de-Almeida MD, Correia F. Metabolic syndrome, adipokines and ghrelin in overweight and obese schoolchildren: results of a 1-year lifestyle intervention programme. Eur J Pediatr. 2011.
16. Verhulst PJ, Depoortere I. Ghrelin's second life: from appetite stimulator to glucose regulator. World J Gastroenterol. 2012.
17. Klok MD, Jakobsdottir S, Drent ML. The role of leptin and ghrelin in the regulation of food intake and body weight in humans: a review. Obes Rev. 2007.
18. Suzuki K, Jayasena CN, Bloom SR. Obesity and appetite control. Exp Diabetes Res. 2012.
19. Wang C, Catlin DH, Starcevic B, Heber D, Ambler C, Berman N, Lucas G, Leung A, Schramm K, Lee PW, Hull L, Swerdloff RS. Low-fat high-fiber diet decreased serum and urine androgens in men. J Clin Endocrinol Metab. 2005.
20. Caronia LM, Dwyer AA, Hayden D, Amati F, Pitteloud N, Hayes FJ. Oral intake of glucose and decrease in Testosterone . Clin Endocrinol (Oxf). 2013.
21. Gardner, et. al. Comparison of the Atkins, Zone, Ornish, and LEARN Diets for Change in Weight and Related Risk Factors Among Overweight Premenopausal Women. JAMA. 2007.
22. Davis, W. Insulin Resistance—A Lethal Link Between Metabolic Disease and Heart Attack. Life Extension Magazine. 2008.

23. IkappaB kinase-beta: NF-kappaB activation and complex formation with I?B kinase-alpha and NIK. Woronicz JD, Gao X, Cao Z, Rothe M, Goeddel DV. 1997, Science, pp. 866–869.

24. The role of superoxide radical in TNF-alpha induced NF-kappaB activation. Wang S, Leonard SS, Castranova V, Vallyathan V, Shi X. 1999, Ann Clin Lab Sci, pp. 192-9.

25. Mohanty P, Hamouda W, Garg R, Aljada A, Ghanim H, Dandona P. 2000, J Clin Endocrinol Metab, pp. 2970-3.

26. Prolonged reactive oxygen species generation and nuclear factor-kappaB activation after a high-fat, high-carbohydrate meal in the obese. Patel C, Ghanim H, Ravishankar S, Sia CL, Viswanathan P, Mohanty P, Dandona P. 2007, J Clin Endocrinol Metab, pp. 4476-9.

27. Dandona P, Aljada A, Bandyopadhyay A. 2004, Trends Immunol., pp. 4-7.

28. Savini I, Catani MV, Evangelista D, Gasperi V, Avigliano L. International Journal of Molecular Sciences.

29. C-reactive protein, interleukin 6, and risk of developing type 2 diabetes mellitus. Pradhan, A.D., et al. 2001, JAMA, pp. 327-34.

30. Forsythe CE, Phinney SD, Fernandez ML, Quann EE, Wood RJ, Bibus DM, Kraemer WJ, Feinman RD, Volek JS. Comparison of low fat and low carbohydrate diets on circulating fatty acid composition and markers of inflammation. Lipids. 2008.

31. Carbohydrate nutrition and inflammatory disease mortality in older adults. Buyken, A.E., et al. 2010, Am J Clin Nutr, pp. 634-43.

32. The association between C-reactive protein levels and insul therapy in obese v. nonobese veterans with type 2 diabetes mellitus. Khatana, S.A., et al. 2010, J Clin Hypertens (Greenwich), pp. 462-8.

33. Goldin, A., et. al. Advanced Glycation End Products. Circulation. 2006.

34. Uribarri. 2007, J Gerontol, pp. 427-33.

35. Effects of low- and high-advanced glycation endproduct meals on macro- and microvascular endothelial function and oxidative stress in patients with type 2 diabetes mellitus. Negrean M, Stirban A, Stratmann B et al. 2007, Am J Clin Nutr, pp. 1236-43.

36. Schinzel, S., et. al. Advanced Glycation End Products and Nutrition. Physiol. Res. 2002.

37. Inflammatory mediators are induced by dietary glycotoxins, a major risk for complications of diabetic angiopathy. Vlassara H, Cai W, Crandall J et al. 2002, Proc Natl Acad Sci.

38. Kellow, N., et. al. Dietary advanced glycation end-product restriction for the attenuation of insulin resistance, oxidative stress and endothelial dysfunction: a systematic review. European Journal of Clinical Nutrition. 2013.

39. Wisse, B. The Inflammatory Syndrome: The Role of Adipose Tissue Cytokines in Metabolic Disorders Due to Obesity. j Am Soc Nephrol. 2004.

40. Calder, P. n-3 Polyunsaturated fatty acids, inflammation, and inflammatory diseases. American Journal of Clinical Nutrition. 2006.

41. Blood Glucose, Insulin, and Diabetes. [Online] http://www.bio.davidson.edu/courses/Bio112/112cp/insdiab.html

42. USDA. http://www.cnpp.usda.gov/Publications/DietaryGuidelines/2010/PolicyDoc/Chapter2.pdf. [Online]

43. Carbohydrate-induced hypertriacylglycerolemia: Historical perspective and review of biological mechanisms. Parks EJ, Hellerstein MK. 2000, Am J Clin Nutr, pp. 412-23.

44. Effect of high-carbohydrate feeding on triglyceride and saturated fatty acid synthesis. LC, Hudgins. 2000, Proc Soc Exp Biol Med, pp. 178-83.

45. Carbohdrate restriction has a more favorable impact on the metabolic syndrome than a low fat diet. Volek, J.S., et al. 2009, Lipids.

46. Is there a simple way to identify insulin resistant individuals at increased risk for cardiovascular disease? McLaughlin, T., et al. 2005, Am J Cardiol, pp. 399-404.

47. The lipid triad in type 2 diabetes—prevalence and relevance of hypertriglyceridaemia/ low high-density lipoprotein syndrome in type 2 diabetes. Temelkova-Kurktschiev T, Hanefeld M. 2004, Exp Clin Endocrinol Diabetes, pp. 75-9.

48. Association of Triglyceride–to–HDL Cholesterol Ratio With Heart Rate Recovery. Shishehbor, et. al. 2004, Diabetes Care, pp. 936-941.

49. Weight loss with a low-carbohydrate, Mediterranean, or low fat diet. Shai, I. et al. 2008, N Engl J Med, pp. 229-41.

50. Metabolic effects of fructose and the worldwide increase in obesity. Tappy L, Lê KA. 2010, Physiol Rev, pp. 23-46.

51. Kordas K, et al. Phytohaemagglutinin inhibits gastric acid but not pepsin secretion in conscious rats. J Physiol Paris. 2001.

52. Pusztai A, et al. Inhibition of starch digestion by alpha-amylase inhibitor reduces the efficiency of utilization of dietary proteins and lipids and retards the growth of rats. J Nutr. 1991.

53. Novel dietary strategy for overcoming the antinutritional effects of soyabean whey of high agglutinin content. . Br J Nutr. . 1997.

54. Ulbricht C, et al. An evidence-based systematic review of stevia by the Natural Standard Research Collaboration. Cardiovasc Hematol Agents Med Chem. 2010.

55. A case of anaphylaxis to erythritol diagnosed by CD203c expression-based basophil activation test. Sugiura S, Kondo Y, Ito K, Hashiguchi A, Takeuchi M, Koyama N. 2013, Annals of allergy, asthma & immunology , pp. 222-223.

56. Bernt WO, et al. Erythritol: a review of biological and toxicological studies. Regul Toxicol Pharmacol. 1996.

57. Abou-Donia MB, et al. Splenda alters gut microflora and increases intestinal p-glycoprotein and cytochrome p-450 in male rats. J Toxicol Environ Health A. 2008.

58. Smith JD, et al. Relief of fibromyalgia symptoms following discontinuation of dietary excitotoxins. Ann Pharmacother. 2001.

59. Stylianos T, et al. he effect of aspartame metabolites on human erythrocyte membrane acetylcholinesterase activity. Pharmacol Res. 2006.

60. Consumption of artificial sweetener- and sugar-containing soda and risk of lymphoma and leukemia in men and women. Am J Clin Nutr. 2012.

61. JH., Lavin. The effect of sucrose- and aspartame-sweetened drinks on energy intake, hunger and food choice of female, moderately restrained eaters. Int J Obes. 1997.

62. Aspartame-fed zebrafish exhibit acute deaths with swimming defects and saccharin-fed zebrafish have elevation of cholesteryl ester transfer protein activity in hypercholesterolemia. Kim JY, Seo J, Cho KH. 2011, Food and chemical toxicology : an international journal published for the British Industrial Biological Research Association, pp. 2899-2905.

63. Healthy intakes of n-3 and n-6 fatty acids: Estimations considering worldwide diversity. Hibbeln, J. R., et al., et al. 2006, The American journal of clinical nutrition.

64. NIH. [Online] http://archive.is/F2eQ.

65. Diets could prevent many diseases. WEM., Lands. 2003, Lipids.

66. Functional foods in primary prevention or nutraceuticals in secondary prevention? WEM., Lands. 2003, Curr Top Nutraceut Res, pp. 113–20.

67. A nation-wide study of atherosclerosis in infants, children and young adults in Japan. Tanaka K, Masuda J, Imamura T, Sueishi K, Nakashima T, Sakurai I, et al. 1988, Atherosclerosis, pp. 143–56.

68. Second nation-wide study of atherosclerosis in infants, children and young adults in Japan. Imakita M, Yutani C, Strong JP, Sakurai I, Sumiyoshi A, Watanabe T, et al. 2001, Atherosclerosis, pp. 487-97.

69. Essential fatty acid requirements in infancy. WFJ., Cuthbertson. 1976, American Journal of Clinical Nutrition, pp. 559–68.

70. Ferreira SH, Moncada S, Vane JR. Indomethacin and aspirin abolish prostaglandin release from the spleen. Nat N Biol. 1971.

71. Lands, WEM. Fish and human health. Orlando : Academic Press, 1986

72. Protective effect of fish oil supplementation on exercise-induced bronchoconstriction in asthma. Mickleborough TD, Lindley MR, Ionescu AA, Fly AD. 2006, Chest, pp. 39–49.

73. Biosynthesis of prostaglandins. WEM., Lands. 1991, Annu Rev Nutr, pp. 41–60.

74. Healthy intakes of n_3 and n_6 fatty acids: estimations considering worldwide diversity. Hibbeln JR, Nieminen LR, Blasbalg TL, Riggs JA, Lands WE. 2006, Am J Clin Nutr, pp. 1483S–93S.

75. Recent concepts on platelet function. Lands WEM, Pitt B, Culp BR. 1980, Herz , pp. 34–41.

76. The effect. Culp BR, Lands WEM, Lucchesi BR, Pitt B, Romson J. 1980, Prostaglandins, pp. 1021–31.

77. Munro IA, Garg ML. Prior supplementation with long chain omega-3 polyunsaturated fatty acids promotes weight loss in obese adults: a double-blinded randomised controlled trial. Food Funct. 2013.

78. Omega-3 fatty acids can be beneficial for joints, helping prevent Rheumatoid arthritis

79. Potent antihypertensive action of dietary flaxseed in hypertensive patients. Rodriguez-Leyva D, Weighell W, Edel AL, Lavallee R, Dibrov E, Pinneker R, Maddaford TG, Ramjiawan B, Aliani M, Guzman R, Pierce GN. 62(6):1081-9, s.l. : Hypertension, December 2013.

80. Omega-3 fatty acids and cardiovascular risk. Kruse LG, Ogletree RL Jr. 54(6):156-7, s.l. : J Miss State Med Assoc, June 2013.

81. This type of heart disease has been associated with low levels of Omega-3 fatty acids

82. Wendel M, Heller AR. Anticancer actions of omega-3 fatty acids--current state and future perspectives. Anticancer Agents Med Chem. 2009.

83. Hibbeln, J. R., L. R. Nieminen, T. L. Blasbalg, J. A. Riggs, W. E. Lands. "Healthy intakes of n_3 and n_6 fatty acids: estimations considering worldwide diversity." Am J Clin Nutr. 2006, pp. 1483S–93S.

84. Effects of winter stocker growth rate and finishing system on: III. Tissue proximate, fatty acid, vitamin and cholesterol content. Duckett, S.K., et al., et al. 2009, Journal of Animal Science, pp. 2961–70.

85. The influence of omega-3 polyunsaturated fatty acids feeding on composition of fatty acids in fatty tissues and eggs of laying hens. Trebunová, A., et al., et al. 2007, Deutsche Tierärztliche Wochenschrift, pp. 275–279.

86. Schirmer MA, Phinney SD. Gamma-linolenate reduces weight regain in formerly obese humans. J Nutr. Jun 2007, pp. 1430-5.

87. Oua, L., et al. Conjugated linoleic acid induces apoptosis of murine mammary tumor cells via Bcl-2 loss. Biochemical and Biophysical Research Communications. 2007, pp. 1044–1049.

88. Whigham LD, Watras AC, Schoeller DA. Efficacy of conjugated linoleic acid for reducing fat mass: a meta-analysis in humans. Am J Clin Nutr. May 2007, pp. 1203-11.

89. Wong JM, de Souza R, Kendall CW, Emam A, Jenkins DJ. Colonic health: fermentation and short chain fatty acids. J Clin Gastroenterol. Mar 2006, pp. 235-43.

90. Di Sabatino A, Morera R, Ciccocioppo R, Cazzola P, Gotti S, Tinozzi FP, Tinozzi S, Corazza GR. Oral butyrate for mildly to moderately active Crohn's disease. Aliment Pharmacol Ther. Nov 1, 2005, pp. 789-94.

91. MEDIUM CHAIN TRIGLYCERIDES (MCTs). [Online] http://www.webmd.com/vitamins-supplements/ingredientmono-915-MEDIUM%20CHAIN%20TRIGLYCERIDES%20%28MCTs%29.aspx?activeIngredientId=915&activeIngredientName=MEDIUM%20CHAIN%20TRIGLYCERIDES%20%28MCTs%29.

92. Hunter, JE., et al. Cardiovascular disease risk of dietary stearic acid compared with trans, other saturated, and unsaturated fatty acids: a systematic review. American Journal of Clinical Nutrition. 2010

93. Dabadie H, Peuchant E, Bernard M, LeRuyet P, Mendy F. Moderate intake of myristic acid in sn-2 position has beneficial lipidic effects and enhances DHA of cholesteryl esters in an interventional study. J Nutr Biochem. Jun 2005, pp. 375-82.

94. RP., Mensink. Effects of stearic acid on plasma lipid and lipoproteins in humans. Lipids. Dec 2005, pp. 1201-5.

95. Wallström, P., et al. Dietary Fiber and Saturated Fat Intake Associations with Cardiovascular Disease Differ by Sex in the Malmö Diet and Cancer Cohort: A Prospective Study. Plos One. 2012.

96. Dashti HM, et al. Long term effects of ketogenic diet in obese subjects with high cholesterol level. Mol Cell Biochem. June 2006.

97. Examining thousands of subjects over a period of decades, the former study director, Dr. William P. Castelli, wrote in the Journal of the American Medical Association: "the more saturated fat one ate, the more cholesterol one ate, the more calories one ate, the lower the person's serum cholesterol."

98. Council., National Research. Fat Content and Composition of Animal Products: Proceedings of a Symposium. Washington, DC : The National Academies Press, 1976.

99. Mansson, H. Fatty acids in bovine milk fat. Food Nutr Res. 2008, p. 52.

100. Circulating oxidised LDL lipids, when proportioned to HDL-c, emerged as a risk factor of all-cause mortality in a population-based survival study. Linna M, Ahotupa M, Lopponen MK, Irjala K, Vasankari T. 2013, Age and ageing, pp. 110-113.

101. Trans fatty acid forming processes in foods: A review. Martin CA, Millinsk MC, Visentainer JV, Matsushita M, De Souza NE. 2007, Anais da Acadmeia Brasileira de Ciencias, pp. 343–350.

102. Kavanagh K, Jones KL, Sawyer J, Kelley K, Carr JJ, Wagner JD, Rudel LL. Trans fat diet induces abdominal obesity and changes in insulin sensitivity in monkeys. Obesity (Silver Spring). 2007, pp. 1675-84.

103. Mensink RP, Katan MB. Effect of dietary trans fatty acids on high-density and low-density lipoprotein cholesterol levels in healthy subjects. N Engl J Med. 1990 .

104. Differential Effects Of Trans And Polyunsaturated Fatty Acids On Ischemia/Reperfusion Injury And Its Associated Cardiovascular Disease States. Ganguly R, Lytwyn MS, Pierce GN. 2013, Current pharmaceutical design.

105. New insights into the health effects of dietary saturated and omega-6 and omega-3 polyunsaturated fatty acids. de Lorgeril M, Salen P. 2012, BMC medicine.

106. Intake of trans fat and all-cause mortality in the Reasons for Geographical and Racial Differences in Stroke (REGARDS) cohort. Kiage JN, Merrill PD, Robinson CJ, et al. 2013, The American journal of clinical nutrition, pp. 1121-1128.

107. Trans fatty acids and cardiovascular health: research completed? Brouwer IA, Wanders AJ, Katan MB. 2013, European journal of clinical nutrition, pp. 541-547.

108. The intake of high fat diet with different trans fatty acid levels differentially induces oxidative stress and non alcoholic fatty liver disease (NAFLD) in rats. Dhibi M, Brahmi F, Mnari A, et al. 2011, Nutrition & metabolism, p. 65.

109. Moderating the portion size of a protein-rich meal improves anabolic efficiency in young and elderly . Symons, et. al. 2009, J Am Diet Assoc, pp. 1582–1586.

110. Institute of Medicine. [Online] [Cited: Nov 27, 2013.] http://www.iom.edu/Global/News%20Announcements/~/media/C5CD2DD7840544979A549EC47E56A02B.ashx.

111. High-protein weight-loss diets: are they afse and do they work? A review of the experimental and epidemiologic data. Eisenstein J, Roberts SB, Dallal G, Saltzman E. 2002, Nutr Rev, pp. 189-200.

112. The significance of protein in food intake and body weight regulation. MS., Westerterp-Plantenga. 2003, Curr Opin Clin Nutr Metab Care, pp. 635–638.

113. Maximal rates of excretion and synthesis of urea in normal and cirrhotic subjects . Rudman D, DiFulco TJ, Galambos JT, Smith RB 3rd, Salam AA, Warren WD. 1973, J Clin Invest, pp. 2241-9.

114. A review of issues of dietary protein intake in humans. Bilsborough, et. al. 2006, Int J Sport Nutr Exerc Metab.

115. Is increased dietary protein necessary or beneficial for individuals with a physically active lifestyle? PW, Lemon. 1996, Nutr Rev, pp. S169-75.

116. Do regular high protein diets have potential health risks on kidney function in athletes? Poortmans JR, Dellalieux O. 2000, Int J Sport Nutr Exerc Metab, pp. 28-38.

117. Dietary protein intake and renal function. Martin WF, Armstrong LE, Rodriguez NR. 2005, Nutr Metab (Lond).

118. Bilsborough, S., N. Mann. "A review of issues of dietary protein intake in humans." Int J Sport Nutr Exerc Metab. 2006, pp. 129–52.

119. Lemon, P. W. "Is increased dietary protein necessary or beneficial for individuals with a physically active lifestyle?" Nutr Rev. 1996, pp. S169–75.

120. Poortmans, J. R., O. Dellalieux. "Do regular high protein diets have potential health risks on kidney function in athletes?" Int J Sport Nutr Exerc Metab. 2000, pp. 28–38.

121. Martin, W. F., L. E. Armstrong, N. R. Rodriguez. "Dietary protein intake and renal function." Nutr Metab (Lond). 2005.

122. Martin, W., et al. "Dietary protein intake and renal function." Nutrition & Metabolism. 2005.

123. Protein and amino acids for athletes. Tipton KD, Wolfe RR. 2004, J Sports Sci, pp. 65-79.

124. Duckett, S. K., J. P. Neel, J. P. Fontenot, W. M. Clapham. "Effects of winter stocker growth rate and finishing system on: III. Tissue proximate, fatty acid, vitamin, and cholesterol content." J Anim Sci. 2009. pp. 2961–70.

125. Ponnampalam EN, Mann NJ, Sinclair AJ. Effect of feeding systems on omega-3 fatty acids, conjugated linoleic acid and trans fatty acids in Australian beef cuts: potential impact on human health. Asia Pac J Clin Nutr. 2006, pp. 21-9.

126. Daley, C., et al. A review of fatty acid profiles and antioxidant content in grass-fed and grain-fed beef. Nutrition Journal. 2010.

127. Descalzo AM, Insani EM, Biolatto A, Sancho AM, García PT, Pensel NA, Josifovich JA. Influence of pasture or grain-based diets supplemented with vitamin E on antioxidant/oxidative balance of Argentine beef. Meat Sci. 2005.

128. Mother Earth News. [Online] 2007. http://www.motherearthnews.com/real-food/tests-reveal-healthier-eggs.aspx#axzz2lnGF5KoE.

129. PCBs in Farmed Salmon. [Online] http://www.ewg.org/research/pcbs-farmed-salmon.

130. Unlabeled Milk From Cows Treated With Biosynthetic Growth Hormones: A Case Of Regulatory Abdication. International Journal of Health Services. 1996.

131. Organo Chlorines and breast cancer Risk by Receptor Status, Tumor Size, and Grade. Cancer Causes and Control (Canada). 2001.

132. Estrogenic Potential of Certain Pyrethroid Compounds in The Mcf-7 Human Breast Carcinoma Cell Line. Environmental Health Perspectives. 1999.

133. HHS. "The Report of the Dietary Guidelines Advisory Committee on Dietary Guidelines for Americans." [Online] http://www.cnpp.usda.gov/dgas2010-dgacreport.htm.

134. The consumption of milk and dairy foods and the incidence of vascular disease and diabetes: an overview of the evidence. Elwood PC, Pickering JE, Givens DI, Gallacher JE. 2010, Lipids, pp. 925–39.

135. Milk and dairy consumption and incidence of cardiovascular diseases and all-cause mortality: dose-response metaanalysis of prospective cohort studies. Soedamah-Muthu SS, Ding EL, Al-Delaimy WK, Hu FB, Engberink MF, WillettWC, Geleijnse JM. 2011, Am J Clin Nutr, pp. 158-71.

136. Dairy consumption and 10-y total and cardiovascular mortality: a prospective cohort study in the Netherlands. Goldbohm RA, Chorus AM, Galindo Garre F, Schouten LJ, van den Brandt PA. 2011, Am J Clin Nutr, pp. 615-27.

137. Major dietary protein sources and risk of coronary heart disease in women. Bernstein AM, Sun Q, Hu FB, Stampfer MJ, Manson JE, Willett WC. 2010, Circulation, pp. 876-83.

138. Soedamah-Muthu, S. S., E. L. Ding, W. K. Al-Delaimy, F. B. Hu, M. F. Engberink, W. C. Willett, J. M. Geleijnse. "Milk and dairy consumption and incidence of cardiovascular diseases and all-cause mortality: dose-response metaanalysis of prospective cohort studies." Am J Clin Nutr. 2011, pp. 158–71.

139. Bernstein AM, Sun Q, Hu FB, Stampfer MJ, Manson JE, Willett WC. 2010, Circulation, pp. 876-83.

140. NIH. Third Report of the National Cholesterol Education Program (NCEP) Expert Panel on: Detection, Evaluation, and Treatment of High Blood Cholesterol in Adults (Adult Treatment Panel III). Final Report. . s.l. : NIH Publications, 2002.

141. Effects of dietary fatty acids and carbohydrates on the ratio of serum total to HDL cholesterol and on serum lipids and apolipoproteins: a meta-analysis of 60 controlled trials. Mensink RP, Zock PL, Kester AD, Katan MB. 2003, Am J Clin Nutr, pp. 1146–55.

142. Saturated fat and cardiometabolic risk factors, coronary heart disease, stroke, and diabetes: a fresh look at the evidence. Micha R, Mozaffarian D. 2010, Lipids, pp. 893-905.

143. Whey protein but not soy protein supplementation alters body weight and composition in free-living overweight and obese adults. Baer DJ, Stote KS, Paul DR, Harris GK, Rumpler WV Clevidence BA. 2011, J Nutr, pp. 1489-1494.

144. If you're not sure this is right for you, consider that a 2008 paper

145. Position of the American Dietetic Association and Dietitians of Canada: Vegetarian diets. 2003, JADA, pp. 748-765.

146. CW., Xiao. Health effects of soy protein and isoflavones in humans. J Nutr. 2008.

147. A review published in 2007 (156) noted that "it does not seem that soy and its constituent isoflavones have met original expectations."

148. Sacks FM, Lichtenstein A, Van Horn L, Harris W, Kris-Etherton P, Winston M and Committee., American Heart Association Nutrition. Soy protein, isoflavones, and cardiovascular health: an American Heart Association Science Advisory for professionals from the Nutrition Committee. Circulation. 2006, pp. 1034-44.

149. Sacks, F., et al. "Soy Protein, Isoflavones, and Cardiovascular Health." Circulation. 2006, pp. 1034–1044 .

150. [Online] http://humrep.oxfordjournals.org/content/23/11/2584.full.

151. Mayer, A. Historical changes in the mineral content of fruits and vegetables. British Food Journal. 1997.

152. Rollo, D., et al. Dietary amelioration of locomotor, neurotransmitter and mitochondrial aging. Exp Biol Med. January 2010

153. Mayer, A. Historical changes in the mineral content of fruits and vegetables. British Food Journal. 1997.

154. GAO. Herbal Dietary Supplements: Examples of Deceptive or Questionable Marketing Practices and Potentially Dangerous Advice. [Online] http://www.gao.gov/products/GAO-10-662T.

155. http://ods.od.nih.gov/factsheets/VitaminD-HealthProfessional/

156. Brøndum-Jacobsen, P, B. G. Nordestgaard, P. Schnohr, and Benn M. "25-hydroxyvitamin D and symptomatic ischemic stroke: an original study and meta-analysis." Ann Neurol. 2013 Jan; 73(1):38–47. Epub 2012 Dec 7. http://www.ncbi.nlm.nih.gov/pubmed/23225498.

157. Pilz, S., W. März, B. Wellnitz, U. Seelhorst, et al. "Association of vitamin D deficiency with heart failure and sudden cardiac death in a large cross-sectional study of patients referred for coronary angiography." Clin Endocrinol Metab. 2008 Oct; 93(10):3927–35. Epub 2008 Aug 5. http://www.ncbi.nlm.nih.gov/pubmed/18682515.

158. Forrest, KY, W. L. Stuhldreher. "Prevalence and correlates of vitamin D deficiency in US adults." Nutr Res. 2011 Jan; 31(1):48–54. http://www.ncbi.nlm.nih.gov/pubmed/21310306

159. Bischoff-Ferrari, HA, W. C. Willett, J. B. Wong, et al. "Fracture prevention with vitamin D supplementation: A meta-analysis of randomized controlled trials." JAMA. 2005; 293(18):2257–2264. http://www.sciencedaily.com/releases/2005/08/050811092620.htm

160. Kongsbak, Martin, Trine B. Levring, Geisler Carsten, Marina Rode von Essen. "The Vitamin D Receptor and T Cell Function." Front Immunol. 2013; 4:148. Published online 2013 June 18. http://www.ncbi.nlm.nih.gov/pmc/articles/PMC3684798/

161. National Institutes of Health. "Calcium, Vitamin D Combo Reduces Bone Loss, Fracture Rate for Older People." NIH News Release. 1997. http://www.nih.gov/news/pr/sept97/nia-03.htm

162. Sitrin, Samuel S., MD. "Vitamin D's role in cell proliferation and differentiation." Nutr Rev. 2008 Oct; 66(10 Suppl 2):S116–24. http://www.ncbi.nlm.nih.gov/pubmed/18844838.

163. Garland, Cedric F., Dr., PH, Frank C. Garland, PhD, Edward D. Gorham, PhD, MPH; et al. "The Role of Vitamin D in Cancer Prevention." Am J Public Health. 2006 February; 96(2):252–261. http://www.ncbi.nlm.nih.gov/pmc/articles/PMC1470481/.

164. Houghton, Lisa A., Reinhold Vieth. "The case against ergocalciferol (vitamin D2) as a vitamin supplement." Am J Clin Nutr. October 2006 vol. 84 no. 4694–697. http://ajcn. nutrition.org/content/84/4/694.full.

165. Coker, Robert H., Sharon Miller, Scott Schutzler, et al. "Whey protein and essential amino acids promote the reduction of adipose tissue and increased muscle protein synthesis during caloric restriction-induced weight loss in elderly, obese individuals." Nutrition Journal. 2012, 11:105. http://www.nutritionj.com/content/11/1/105.

166. Bounous, G, G. Batist, P. Gold, "Immunoenhancing property of dietary whey protein in mice: role of glutathione." Clin Invest Med. 1989 Jun; 12(3):154–61. http://www.ncbi. nlm.nih.gov/pubmed/2743633.

167. Frid, A. H., M. Nilsson, J. J. Holst, et al. "Effect of whey on blood glucose and insulin responses to composite breakfast and lunch meals in type 2 diabetic subjects." Am J Clin Nutr. 2005 Jul; 82(1):69–75. http://www.ncbi.nlm.nih.gov/pubmed/16002802.

168. Davis, J. M., E. A. Murphy, M. D. Carmichael, M. R. Zielinski, C. M. Groschwitz, A. S. Brown, A. Ghaffar, E. P. Mayer. "Curcumin effects on inflammation and performance recovery following eccentric exercise-induced muscle damage." Am J Physiol Regul Integr Comp Physiol. 2007 Mar 1. http://umm.edu/health/medical/altmed/herb/turmeric.

169. Thakur, C. P., B. Thakur, S. Singh, et al. "The Ayurvedic medicines Haritaki, Amala and Bahira reduce cholesterol-induced atherosclerosis in rabbits." Int J Cardiol. 1988 Nov; 21(2):167–75. http://www.ncbi.nlm.nih.gov/pubmed/3225068.

170. http://www.mayoclinic.com/health/toxic-hepatitis/DS00811/DSECTION=causes

171. Loomis, Dana, Yann Grosse, Beatrice Lauby-Secretan, et al. "The carcinogenicity of outdoor air pollution." The Lancet Oncology. Vol. 14 No. 13 pp 1262–1263. http://www. thelancet.com/journals/lanonc/article/PIIS1470-2045%2813%2970487-X/fulltext

172. Manifestations of Toxic Effects. http://pmep.cce.cornell.edu/profiles/extoxnet/TIB/manifestations.html

173. Rankin, Lucille C., Joanna R. Groom, Michael Chopin, et al. "The transcription factor T-bet is essential for the development of NKp46+ innate lymphocytes via the Notch pathway." Nature Immunology. 14,389–395, (2013). http://www.nature.com/ni/journal/v14/n4/abs/ni.2545.html.

174. Park, Sung Kyun, Katherine L. Tucker, Marie S. O'Neill, et al. "Fruit, vegetable, and fish consumption and heart rate variability: the Veterans Administration Normative Aging Study." Am J Clin Nutr. March 2009, vol. 89 no. 3778–786. http://ajcn.nutrition.org/content/89/3/778.

175. Parker, G., N. A. Gibson, H. Brotchie, et al. "Omega-3 fatty acids and mood disorders." Am J Psychiatry. 2006 Jun; 163(6):969–78. http://www.ncbi.nlm.nih.gov/pubmed/16741195.

176. Teague, H., Cassie Fhaner, Mitchel Harris, et al. "N-3 PUFAs enhance the frequency of murine B cell subsets and restore the impairment of antibody production to a T-independent antigen in obesity." J Lipid Res. 2013 Nov; 54(11):3130–8. doi: 10.1194/jlr.M042457. http://www.ncbi.nlm.nih.gov/pubmed/23986558.

177. Maroon, J. C., J. W. Bost. "Omega-3 fatty acids (fish oil) as an anti-inflammatory: an alternative to nonsteroidal anti-inflammatory drugs for discogenic pain." Surg Neurol. 2006 Apr; 65(4):326–31. http://www.ncbi.nlm.nih.gov/pubmed/16531187.

178. Kiecolt-Glaser, Janice K., Martha A. Belury, Rebecca Andridge, et al. "Omega-3 supplementation lowers inflammation and anxiety in medical students: A randomized controlled trial." Brain, Behavior, and Immunity. 2011. http://www.sciencedirect.com/science/article/pii/S0889159111004685.

179. Simopoulos, A. P. "The importance of the ratio of omega-6/omega-3 essential fatty acids." Biomed Pharmacother. 2002 Oct; 56(8):365–79. http://www.ncbi.nlm.nih.gov/pubmed/12442909.

180. http://www.thorne.com/altmedrev/.fulltext/9/1/70.pdf

181. Emory University. "Beneficial bacteria help repair intestinal injury by inducing reactive oxygen species." ScienceDaily. May 11, 2011; Retrieved December 18, 2013. Error! Hyperlink reference not valid.

182. Paur, I., T. R. Balstad, M. Kolberg, et al. "Extract of oregano, coffee, thyme, clove, and walnuts inhibits NF-kappaB in monocytes and in transgenic reporter mice." Cancer Prev Res (Phila). 2010 May; 3(5): 653–63. doi: 10.1158/1940-6207.CAPR-09-0089. Epub 2010 Apr 27. http://www.ncbi.nlm.nih.gov/pubmed/20424131.

183. Fu Y., Y. Zu Y, L. Chen, X. Shi, Z. Wang, S. Sun, T. Efferth. "Antimicrobial activity of clove and rosemary essential oils alone and in combination." Phytother Res. 2007 Oct; 21(10):989–94. PMID: 17562569. http://www.ncbi.nlm.nih.gov/pubmed/17562569.

184. Du, W. X., C. W. Olsen, R. J. Avena-Bustillos, et al. "Antibacterial effects of allspice, garlic, and oregano essential oils in tomato films determined by overlay and vapor-phase methods." J Food Sci. 2009Sep; 74(7):M390–7. http://www.ncbi.nlm.nih.gov/pubmed/19895486

185. Nzeako, B. C., Z. S. N. Al-Kharousi, Z. Al-Mahrooqui. "Antimicrobial Activities of Clove and Thyme Extracts." Sultan Qaboos Univ Med J. 2006 June; 6(1):33–39. http://www.ncbi.nlm.nih.gov/pmc/articles/PMC3074903/

186. USDA. http://ndb.nal.usda.gov/ndb/search/list. [Online]

187. USDA. http://ndb.nal.usda.gov/ndb/search/list. [Online]

188. AJCN. [Online] http://ajcn.nutrition.org/content/76/1/5.full.pdf.

189. Samaha, F., et al. A Low-Carbohydrate as Compared with a Low-Fat Diet in Severe Obesity. N Engl J Med. 2003.

190. Yancy WS Jr, Olsen MK, Guyton JR, Bakst RP, Westman EC. A low-carbohydrate, ketogenic diet versus a low-fat diet to treat obesity and hyperlipidemia: a randomized, controlled trial. Ann Intern Med. 2004.

191. Shai, I., et al. Weight Loss with a Low-Carbohydrate, Mediterranean, or Low-Fat Diet. N Engl J Med. 2008.

192. Krebs, N., et al. Efficacy and Safety of a High Protein, Low Carbohydrate Diet for Weight Loss in Severely Obese Adolescents. Journal of Pediatrics. 2010.

193. Howard, BV, et al. Low-fat dietary pattern and weight change over 7 years: the Women's Health Initiative Dietary Modification Trial. JAMA. 2006.

194. Low-Fat Dietary Pattern and Risk of Cardiovascular Disease. JAMA. 2006.

195. Prentice RL, et. al. Low-fat dietary pattern and risk of invasive breast cancer: the Women's Health Initiative Randomized Controlled Dietary Modification Trial. JAMA. 2006.

196. Health.gov. [Online] http://www.health.gov/dietaryguidelines/dga2005/report/HTML/G5_History.htm

197. Brillat-Savarin, J. The Physiology of Taste. Somerset : The Heritage Press, 1949.

198. Spock, B. Baby and Child Care. New York City : s.n., 1945

199. Time. Jan. 13, 1961

200. YERUSHALMY J, HILLEBOE HE. Fat in the diet and mortality from heart disease; a methodologic note. N Y State J Med. 1957.

201. Krieger, J., et al. Effects of variation in protein and carbohydrate intake on body mass and composition during energy restriction: a meta-regression. American Journal of Clinical Nutrition. [Online]

202. Ludwig, D, Ebbeling, C, et al. Effects of Dietary Composition on Energy Expenditure During Weight-Loss Maintenance. JAMA. 2012.

203. Srikanthan, P., Karlamangla, A. Relative Muscle Mass Is Inversely Associated with Insulin Resistance and Prediabetes. Findings from The Third National Health and Nutrition Examination Survey. The Journal of Clinical Endocrinology & Metabolism. 2011.

204. Effect of high-carbohydrate feeding on triglyceride and saturated fatty acid synthesis. LC., Hudgins. 2000, Proc Soc Exp Biol Med, pp. 178-83.

205. Santos FL, Esteves SS, da Costa Pereira A, Yancy WS Jr, Nunes JP. Systematic review and meta-analysis of clinical trials of the effects of low carbohydrate diets on cardiovascular risk factors. Obes Rev. 2012.

206. Shai, I., et al. "Weight Loss with a low carbohydrate, Mediterranean, or Low-Fat Diet." N Engl J Med. 2008.

207. Brehm, B., et al. "A Randomized Trial Comparing a Very Low Carbohydrate Diet and a Calorie-Restricted Low Fat Diet on Body Weight and Cardiovascular Risk Factors in Healthy Women." The Journal of Clinical Endocrinology & Metabolism. 2003.

208. Samaha, et al. "A low carbohydrate as Compared with a Low-Fat Diet in Severe Obesity." N Engl J Med. 2003.

209. Krebs, N., et al. "Efficacy and Safety of a High Protein, Low Carbohydrate Diet for Weight Loss in Severely Obese Adolescents." The Journal of Pediatrics. 2010.

210. Sondike, S., et al. "Effects of a low carbohydrate diet on weight loss and cardiovascular risk factor in overweight adolescents." The Journal of Pediatrics. March 2003, pp. 253–258.

211. Westman, E., et al. "The effect of a low carbohydrate, ketogenic diet versus a low-glycemic index diet on glycemic control in type 2 diabetes mellitus." Nutrition & Metabolism. 2008.

212. Keogh, J., et al. "Effects of weight loss from a very-low carbohydrate diet on endothelial function and markers of cardiovascular disease risk in subjects with abdominal obesity." Am J Clin Nutr. Mar 2008, pp. 567–576 .

213. Brinkworth, G. D., M. Noakes, J. D. Buckley, J. B. Keogh, P. M. Clifton. "Long-term effects of a very-low carbohydrate weight loss diet compared with an isocaloric low-fat diet after 12 mo." Am J Clin Nutr. 2009.

214. Brehm, B., et al. "The Role of Energy Expenditure in the Differential Weight Loss in Obese Women on Low-Fat and low carbohydrate Diets." The Journal of Clinical Endocrinology & Metabolism. 2005.

215. Gardner, C., et al. "Comparison of the Atkins, Zone, Ornish, and LEARN Diets for Change in Weight and Related Risk Factors Among Overweight Premenopausal Women." JAMA. 2007.

216. Feinman, R. D., J. S. Volek. "Low carbohydrate diets improve atherogenic dyslipidemia even in the absence of weight loss." Nutr Metab (Lond). Jun 2006.

217. Severe NAFLD with hepatic necroinflammatory changes in mice fed trans fats and a high-fructose corn syrup equivalent. Tetri LH, Basaranoglu M, Brunt EM, Yerian LM, Neuschwander-Tetri. 295(5):G987-995, s.l. : American journal of gastrointestinal and liver physiology, 2008.

218. Schultz, A., D. Neil D, M. B. Aguila, C. A. Mandarim-de-Lacerda. "Hepatic adverse effects of fructose consumption independent of overwight/obesity." 14(11):21873–21886, s.l. : International journal of molecular sciences. 2013.

219. Hu, F. B. "Resolved: there is sufficient scientific evidence that decreasing sugar-sweetened beverage consumption will reduce the prevalence of obesity and obesity-related diseases." 14(8):606–619, s.l. : Obesity reviews: an official journal of the International Association for the Study of Obesity. 2013.

220. Association between sucrose intake and cancer: a review of the evidence. Aranceta Bartrina J, Perez Rodrigo C. Suppl 4:95-105, s.l. : Nuticion hospitalaria, 2013.

221. Sugars in diet and risk of cancer in the NIH-AARP Diet and Health Study. Tasevska N, Jiao L, Cross AJ, et al. 130(1):159-169, s.l. : International Journal of cancer, 2012.

222. Taubes, G. Is Sugar Toxic? New York Times. 2011.

223. Fructose and metabolic diseases: new findings, new questions. Tappy L, Le KA, Tran C, Paquot N. 26(11-12):1044-1049, Burbank, California : Nutrition, 2012.

224. Wang C, Catlin DH, Starcevic B, Heber D, Ambler C, Berman N, Lucas G, Leung A, Schramm K, Lee PW, Hull L, Swerdloff RS. Low-fat high-fiber diet decreased serum and urine androgens in men. J Clin Endocrinol Metab. 2005.

225. Caronia LM, Dwyer AA, Hayden D, Amati F, Pitteloud N, Hayes FJ. Abrupt decrease in serum testosterone levels after an oral glucose load in men: implications for screening for hypogonadism. Clin Endocrinol (Oxf). 2013.

226. Fry AC, Lohnes CA. Acute testosterone and cortisol responses to high power resistance exercise. Fiziol Cheloveka. 2010.

227. Pilz S, Frisch S, Koertke H, Kuhn J, Dreier J, Obermayer-Pietsch B, Wehr E, Zittermann A. Effect of vitamin D supplementation on testosterone levels in men. Horm Metab Res. 2011.

228. Chronically-high levels of cortisol can lead to the loss of lean muscle tissue

229. A 2010 study demonstrated that low-calorie dieting increases cortisol

230. Weigensberg MJ, Lane CJ, Winners O, Wright T, Nguyen-Rodriguez S, Goran MI, Spruijt-Metz D. Acute effects of stress-reduction Interactive Guided Imagery(SM) on salivary cortisol in overweight Latino adolescents. J Altern Complement Med. 2009.

231. Kanai, et. al. Huggable communication medium decreases cortisol levels. Sci Rep. 2013.

232. Zeisel, et. al. Dose Response Effects of Dermally applied Diethanolamine on Neurogenesis in Fetal Mouse Hippocampus and Potential Exposure of Humans . Toxicol. Sci. 2009.

233. Contribution of leptin receptor N-linked glycans to leptin binding. Kamikubo Y, Dellas C, Loskutoff DJ, Quigley JP, Ruggeri ZM. 2008, Biochem J.

234. Prevention and reversal of diet-induced leptin resistance with a sugar-free diet despite high fat content. Shapiro A, Tümer N, Gao Y, Cheng KY, Scarpace PJ. 2011, Br J Nutr.

235. Triglycerides induce leptin resistance at the blood-brain barrier. Banks WA, Coon AB, Robinson SM, Moinuddin A, Shultz JM, Nakaoke R, Morley JE. 2004, Diabetes, pp. 1253-60.

236. Medline Plus. [Online] http://www.nlm.nih.gov/medlineplus/vitamina.html

237. Medline Plus. [Online] http://www.nlm.nih.gov/medlineplus/ency/article/002405.htm

238. NIH. [Online] http://ods.od.nih.gov/factsheets/VitaminE-HealthProfessional/

239. MedLine Plus. [Online] http://www.nlm.nih.gov/medlineplus/ency/article/002407.htm

240. MedLine Plus. [Online] http://www.nlm.nih.gov/medlineplus/ency/article/002411.htm

241. WebMD. [Online] http://www.webmd.com/vitamins-and-supplements/lifestyle-guide-11/supplement-guide-niacin.

242. NIH. [Online] http://ods.od.nih.gov/factsheets/VitaminB6-HealthProfessional/.

243. MedLine Plus. [Online] http://www.nlm.nih.gov/medlineplus/druginfo/natural/313.html

244. NIH. [Online] http://ods.od.nih.gov/factsheets/Folate-HealthProfessional

245. NIH. [Online] http://ods.od.nih.gov/factsheets/VitaminB12-QuickFacts/.

246. WebMD. [Online] http://www.webmd.com/food-recipes/guide/vitamins-and-minerals-good-food-sources.

247. al, Lee et. 2005, JAMA, pp. 56-65.

248. Haines ST, Park SK. Vitamin D supplementation: what's known, what to do, and what's needed. Pharmacotherapy. 2012.

249. Vitamin D: importance in the prevention of cancers, type 1 diabetes, heart disease, and osteoporosis. Holick, M. 2004, American Journal of Clinical Nutrition.

250. independent association of low serum 25-hydroxyvitamin D and 1, 25-dihyddroxyvitamin D levels with all-cause and cardiovascular mortality. Dobnig H, et al. Arch Intern Med, pp. 1340-9.

251. NIH. [Online] http://www.nlm.nih.gov/medlineplus/ency/article/002401.htm.

252. NIH. [Online] http://www.nlm.nih.gov/medlineplus/ency/article/002411.htm

253. Institute of Medicine. [Online] http://www.iom.edu/Global/News%20Announcements/~/media/474B28C39EA34C43A60A6D42CCE07427.ashx.

254. Takanami Y, Iwane H, Kawai Y, Shimomitsu T. Vitamin E supplementation and endurance exercise: are there benefits? Sports Med. 2000.

255. Vitamin E and vitamin C supplement use and risk of all-cause and coronary heart disease mortality in older persons: the established populations for epidemiological studies of the elderly. Losonczy KG, et al. 1996, Amer J Clin Nutr, pp. 190-6.

256. FH., Nielsen. Magnesium, inflammation, and obesity in chronic disease. Nutr Rev. 2010.

257. External influences on the fetus and their long-term consequences. DIW., Phillips. 2006, Lupus, pp. 794-800.

258. Epigenetic regulation of fetal bone development and placental transfer of nutrients: Progress for osteoporosis. Bocheva G, et al. 2011, Interdiscip Toxicol, pp. 167-2.

259. Nutrition in pregnancy: Mineral and vitamin supplements. OA., Ldipo. 2000, Am J Clin Nutr.

260. Maternal Nutrition and Fetal Development. Spencer, et. al. 2004, J. Nutr., pp. 2169-2172.

261. Hacker, N., Moore, J.G., & Gambone, J.C. Essentials of Obstetrics and Gynecology (4th ed.). Philadelphia : Saunders, 2004.

262. Rasumssen KM, Yaktine AL. Weight Gain During Pregnancy: Reexamining the Guidelines. Washington, DC : s.n., 2009.

263. Worthington-Roberts, B.S., & Williams, S.R. Nutrition in Pregnancy and Lactation (6th ed.). Dubuque : McGraw-Hill, 1997.

264. Energy, Carbohydrate, Fiber, Fatty Acids, Cholesterol, Protein, and Amino Acids: Dietary Reference Intakes. Washington, DC : National Academies Press, 2002.

265. Dietary Reference Intakes for Energy, Carbohydrate, Fiber, Fat, Fatty Acids, Cholesterol, Protein, and Amino Acids. Washington, DC : National Academy Press, 2002.

266. A comparative evaluation of vegan, vegetarian, and omnivore diets. Carlson E, et al. 1985, J Plant Foods, pp. 89-100.

267. The recommended dietary allowances (RDAs) for folate are as follows

268. Council, National Research. Dietary Reference Intakes for Thiamin, Riboflavin, Niacin, Vitamin B6, Folate, Vitamin B12, Pantothenic Acid, Biotin, and Choline. Washington, DC : The National Academies Press, 1998.

269. Food and Nutrition Board. Dietary Reference Intakes for Vitamin A, Vitamin K, Arsenic, Boron, Chromium, Copper, Iodine, Iron, Manganese, Molybdenum, Nickel, Silicon, Vanadium, and Zinc. Washington, DC : National Academy Press, 2001.

270. Vitamin D deficiency during pregnancy: An ongoing epidemic. Hollis BW, et al. 2006, Am J Clin Nutr, pp. 350-3.

271. Vitamin D and calcium supplementation reduces cancer risk: results of a randomized trial. 2007, Am J Clin Nutr, pp. 1586-1591.

272. Association between Residences in U.S. Northern Latitudes and Rheumatoid Arthritis: A Spatial Analysis of the Nurses' Health Study. al., Vieira et. 2010, Environmental Health Perspectives.

273. Assessment of iron status in U.S. pregnant women from the National Health and Nutrition Examination Survey (NHANES). Mei Z, et al. 2011, Am J Clin Nutr, pp. 1312-20.

274. Another element to pay attention to is iodine. You don't need a lot of iodine on a daily basis, but its presence is required for normal thyroid function, which helps foster the ideal physical and mental growth of the baby

275. Scholtz SA, Colombo J, Carlson SE. Clinical Overview of Effects of Dietary Long-Chain Polyunsaturated Fatty Acids during the Perinatal Period. Lawrence, KS : s.n.

276. Towards establishing dietary reference intakes for eicosapentaenoic and docosahexaenoic acids. Harris WS, et al. 2009, J Nutr, pp. 804S-19S.

277. Assessing Omega-3 Fatty Acid Supplementation During Pregnancy and Lactation to Optimize Maternal Mental Health and Childhood Cognitive Development. Klemens, et. al. 2012, Lipidology, pp. 93-109.

278. Fetal and Neonatal Levels of Omega-3: Effects on Neurodevelopment, Nutrition, and Growth. Bernardi, et. al. 2012, The Scientific World Journal.

279. Visual acuity and cognitive outcomes at 4 years of age in a double-blind, randomized trial of long-chain polyunsaturated fatty acid-supplemented infant formula. irch EE, Garfield S, Castaneda Y, et al. 2007, Early Hum Dev., pp. 279-84.

280. Maternal fatty acid status during pregnancy and lactation and relation to newborn and infant status. Lauritzen L, Carlson SE. 2011, Matern Child Nutr, pp. 41-58.

281. Position of the American Dietetic Association: Promoting and supporting breastfeeding. James DC, et al. 2009, J Am Diet Assoc., pp. 1926–42.

282. The burden of suboptimal breastfeeding in the United States: A pediatric cost analysis. Bartick M, et al. 2010, Pediatrics, pp. e1048-56.

283. Breastfeeding and the risk of childhood acute leukemia. Shu X-O, et al. 1999, J Natl Cancer Inst, pp. 1765-72.

284. An Exploratory Study of Environmental and Medical Factors Potentially Related to Childhood Cancer. 1991, Medical & Pediatric Oncology, pp. 115-21.

285. Perinatal Characteristics and risk of rheumatoid arthritis. al, Jacobsson LTH et. 2003, BMJ, pp. 1068-1069.

286. A prospective cohort study on breast-feeding and otitis media in Swedish infants. Aniansson G, Alm B, Andersson B, et al. 1994, Pediatr Infect Dis J, pp. 183-188.

287. The association between duration of breastfeeding and adult intelligence. al, Mortensen EL et. 2002, JAMA, pp. 2365-71.

288. Breastfeeding and cognitive development: a meta-analysis. al, Anderson JW et. 1999, Am J Clin Nutr, pp. 525-3.

289. Breast feeding and respiratory morbidity in infancy: a birth cohort study. Oddy, WH et al. 2003, Archives of Disease in Childhood, pp. 224-228.

290. Breastfeeding and the Risk of Hospitalization for Respiratory Disease in Infancy. al, Galton Bachrach et. 2003, Arch Pediatr Adolesc Med, pp. 237-243.

291. Epidemiology of acute diarrheal diseases in children in a high standard of living settlement in Israel. Lerman, Y. et al. 1994, Pediatr Infect Dis J, pp. 116-22.

292. Association between breast feeding and asthma in 6 year old children: findings of a prospective birth cohort study. Burton, et. al. 1999, BMJ.

293. Long-term effects of the intrauterine environment, birth weight, and breast-feeding in Pima Indians. Pettitt DJ, Knowler WC. 1998, Diabetes Care, pp. B138-41.

294. Breast-feeding and the risk of breast cancer in BRCA1 and BRCA2 mutation carriers. Jernstrom, H et al. 2004, J Natl Cancer Inst, pp. 1094-1098.

295. Effect of lifetime lactation on breast cancer risk: a Korean women's cohort study. Lee, SY et al. 2003, Int J Cancer, pp. 390-393.

296. Lactation and a reduced risk of premenopausal breast cancer. Newcomb PA, Storer BE, Longnecker MP, et al. 1994, N Engl J Med, pp. 81-87.

297. Institute of Medicine. [Online] http://www.iom.edu/Global/News%20 Announcements/~/media/C5CD2DD7840544979A549EC47E56A02B.ashx.

298. PJ., Garlick. Protein requirements of infants and children. 2006.

299. Health.gov. [Online] http://www.health.gov/dietaryguidelines/dga2005/report/HTML/table_d3_1.htm

300. Estelle V. Lambert, David P. Speechly, Steven C. Dennis, Timothy D. Noakes. Enhanced endurance in trained cyclists during moderate intensity exercise following 2 weeks adaption to a high fat diet. European Journal of Applied Physiology and Occupational Physiology. 1994.

301. Langfort J, Pilis W, Zarzeczny R, Nazar K, Kaciuba-Uścitko H. Effect of low-carbohydrate-ketogenic diet on metabolic and hormonal responses to graded exercise in men. Department of Applied Physiology Medical Research Centre. 1996.

302. The human metabolic response to chronic ketosis without caloric restriction: Preservation of submaximal exercise capability with reduced carbohydrate oxidation. Metabolism. 1983.

303. R, Bahr. Excess postexercise oxygen consumption--magnitude, mechanisms and practical implications. Acta Physiologica Scandinavica. 1992.

304. Phelian, J.F, Reinke, E., Harris, M.A. and Melby, C.L. Post-exercise energy expenditure and substrate oxidation in young women resulting from exercise bouts of different intensity. Journal of the American College of Nutrition. 1997.

305. Bielinski R, Schutz Y, Jéquier E. Energy metabolism during the postexercise recovery in man. The American Journal of Clinical Nutrition.

306. Borsheim, E. and Bahr, R. Effect of exercise intensity, duration and mode on post-exercise oxygen consumption. Sports Medicine. 2003.

307. LaForgia, J., Withers, R.T., & Gore, C.J. Effects of exercise intensity and duration on the excess post-exercise oxygen consumption. . J. Sports Sci. 2006

308. Effect of exercise on recovery changes in plasma levels of FFA, glycerol, glucose and catecholamines. Scandinavian Physiological Society. 1991.

309. Little JP, Safdar A, Bishop D, Tarnopolsky MA, Gibala MJ. An acute bout of high-intensity interval training increases the nuclear abundance of PGC-1α and activates mitochondrial biogenesis in human skeletal muscle. Am J Physiol Regul Integr Comp Physiol. 2011.

310. Gibala, M. Molecular responses to high-intensity interval exercise. Applied Physiology, Nutrition, and Metabolism. 2009.

311. Burgomaster, K.A., et al. Similar metabolic adaptations during exercise after low volume sprint interval and traditional endurance training in humans. Journal of Physiology. 2008.

312. Pesta, D., et al. Similar qualitative and quantitative changes of mitochondrial respiration following with strength and endurance training in normoxia and hypoxia in sedentary humans. Integrative and Comparative Physiology. 2011.

313. Horowitz, et. al. Lipolytic suppression following carbohydrate ingestion limits fat oxidation during exercise. J Appl Physiol. 2009.

314. Hopper, et. al. Exercise metabolism at different time intervals after a meal. J of Applied Physiology. 1991.

315. Cappon JP, Ipp E, Brasel JA, Cooper DM. Acute effects of high fat and high glucose meals on the growth hormone response to exercise. J Clin Endocrinol Metab. 1993.

316. Berardi, J. M., Price, T. B., Noreen, E. E., and Lemon, P. W. Postexercise muscle glycogen recovery enhanced with a carbohydrate-protein supplement. Medicine and Science in Sports and Exercise. 2006.

317. Rasmussen, B.B., K.D. Tipton, S.L. Miller, S.E. Wolf, and R.R. Wolfe. An oral essential amino acid-carbohydrate supplement enhances muscle protein anabolism after resistance exercise. J. Appl. Physiol. 2000.

318. Andersen, et. al. Timing of postexercise protein intake is important for muscle hypertrophy with resistance training in elderly humans. The Journal of Physiology. 2001.

319. Pennings, B., Koopman, R., Beelen, M., et al. Exercising before protein intake allows for greater use of protein-derived amino acids for de novo muscle protein synthesis in both young and elderly mrn. American Journal of Clinical Nutrition. 2011.

320. Tipton, K.D., T.A. Elliott, M.G. Cree, S.E. Wolf, A.P. Sanford, and R.R. Wolfe. Ingestion of casein and whey proteins result in muscle anabolism after resistance exercise. Med. Sci. Sports Exerc. 2004.

321. Langenfeld ME, Seifert JG, Rudge SR, Bucher RJ. Effect of carbohydrate ingestion on performance of non-fasted cyclists during a simulated 80-mile time trial. J Sports Med Phys Fitness. 1994.

322. The standard rule of thumbs for carbohydrates and hydration during exercise, as indicated by the International Society of Sports Nutrition

323. Kalman, et. al. Comparison of coconut water and a carbohydrate-electrolyte sport drink on measures of hydration and physical performance in exercise-trained men. Journal of the International Society of Sports Nutrition. 2012.

324. Ismail I, Singh R, Sirisinghe RG. Rehydration with sodium-enriched with sodium-enriched coconut water after exercise-induced dehydration. Southeast Asian J Trop Med Public Health. 2007

325. Saat, R. Singh, R. Sirissinghe, M. Nawawi. Rehydration after Exercise with Fresh Young Coconut Water, Carbohydrate-Electrolyte Beverage and Plain Water. Journal of Physiology and Anthropology and Applied Human Science. 2002.

326. Consensus Statement of the 1st International Exercise-Associated Hyponatremia Consensus Development Conference. Clinical Journal of Sport Medicine. 2005.

327. Dietary Reference Intakes for Water, Sodium, Cholride, Potassium and Sulfate. Washington DC : National Academy Press, 2005.

328. Lopez, A., et al. Global and regional burden of disease and risk factors, 2001: systematic analysis of population health data. The Lancet. 2006, pp. 1747-57.

329. Vasanthi HR, Parameswari RP, DeLeiris J, Das DK. Health benefits of wine and alcohol from neuroprotection to heart health. Front Biosci (Elite Ed). 2012, pp. 1505-12.

330. Blackhurst, D., et al. Alcohol: foe or friend? South African Medical Journal. 2005.

331. Britton A, Marmot MG, Shipley M. Who benefits most from the cardioprotective properties of alcohol consumption--health freaks or couch potatoes? J Epidemiol Community Health. 2008, pp. 905-8.

332. Rimm EB, Klatsky A, Grobbee D, Stampfer MJ. Review of moderate alcohol consumption and reduced risk of coronary heart disease: is the effect due to beer, wine, or spirits. British Medical Journal. 1996.

333. French MT, Zavala SK. The health benefits of moderate drinking revisited: alcohol use and self-reported health status. Am J Health Promot. 2007.

334. WebMD. [Online] http://www.webmd.com/diet/features/the-truth-about-seven-common-food-additives.

335. Ciardi C, Jenny M, Tschoner A, Ueberall F, Patsch J, Pedrini M, Ebenbichler C, Fuchs D. Food additives such as sodium sulphite, sodium benzoate and curcumin inhibit leptin release in lipopolysaccharide-treated murine adipocytes in vitro. Br J Nutr. 2012, pp. 826-33.

336. Phys.org. [Online] http://phys.org/news183110037.html.

337. Better Health Channel. [Online] http://www.betterhealth.vic.gov.au/bhcv2/bhcarticles.nsf/pages/Food_additives.

338. National Resources Defense Council. [Online] http://www.nrdc.org/water/drinking/uscities.asp

339. National Resources Defense Council. [Online] http://www.nrdc.org/health/effects/mercury/guide.asp

340. CDC. [Online] http://www.cdc.gov/nceh/lead/tips.htm.

341. Sanderson W.T., Talaska G, Zaebst D, et al. Pesticide prioritization for a brain cancer case control study. Environ Res. 1997.

342. Grinder-Pederson L, Rasmussen SE, Bugel S, et al. Worthington V. Nutritional quality of organic versus conventional fruits, vegetables and grains. J Alt Coml Med. 2001.

343. Blom, et. al. Effect of a high-protein breakfast on the postprandial ghrelin response. Am J Clin Nutr. 2006.

344. Buckley JD, Howe PR. Long chain omega 3 polyunsaturated fatty acids may be beneficial for reducing obesity. Nutrients. 2010.

345. Forsythe CE, Phinney SD, Fernandez ML, Quann EE, Wood RJ, Bibus DM, Kraemer WJ, Feinman RD, Volek JS. Comparison of low fat and low carbohydrate diets on circulating fatty acid composition and markers of inflammation. Lipids. 2008.

About the Author

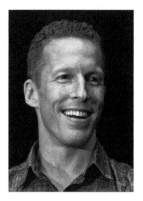

Dr. Ben Lerner is the co-founder of Maximized Living, Maximized Living Health Centers, and the Maximized Living Foundation. He has owned and operated five clinics in Central Florida. These clinics cared for over 12,000 total patients each month with a combination of pediatric, wellness care, corrective care, sports performance, personal injury, and a special attention to chronic illness.

Dr. Lerner is currently the co-chairman for the Sports Performance Council that provides care for many of the U.S. sports governing bodies as well as with teams and athletes at the professional, collegiate, and high school levels.

He is the author of ten books and has spent multiple weeks on the New York Times, Wall Street Journal, and USA Today Best Sellers lists. He lives in Celebration, Fla., with his wife Dr. Sheri Lerner and their three children, Skylar, Nicole, and Cael.